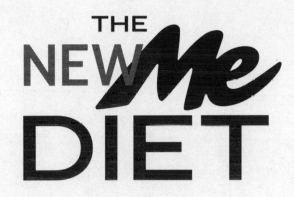

THE NEW **Me** DIET

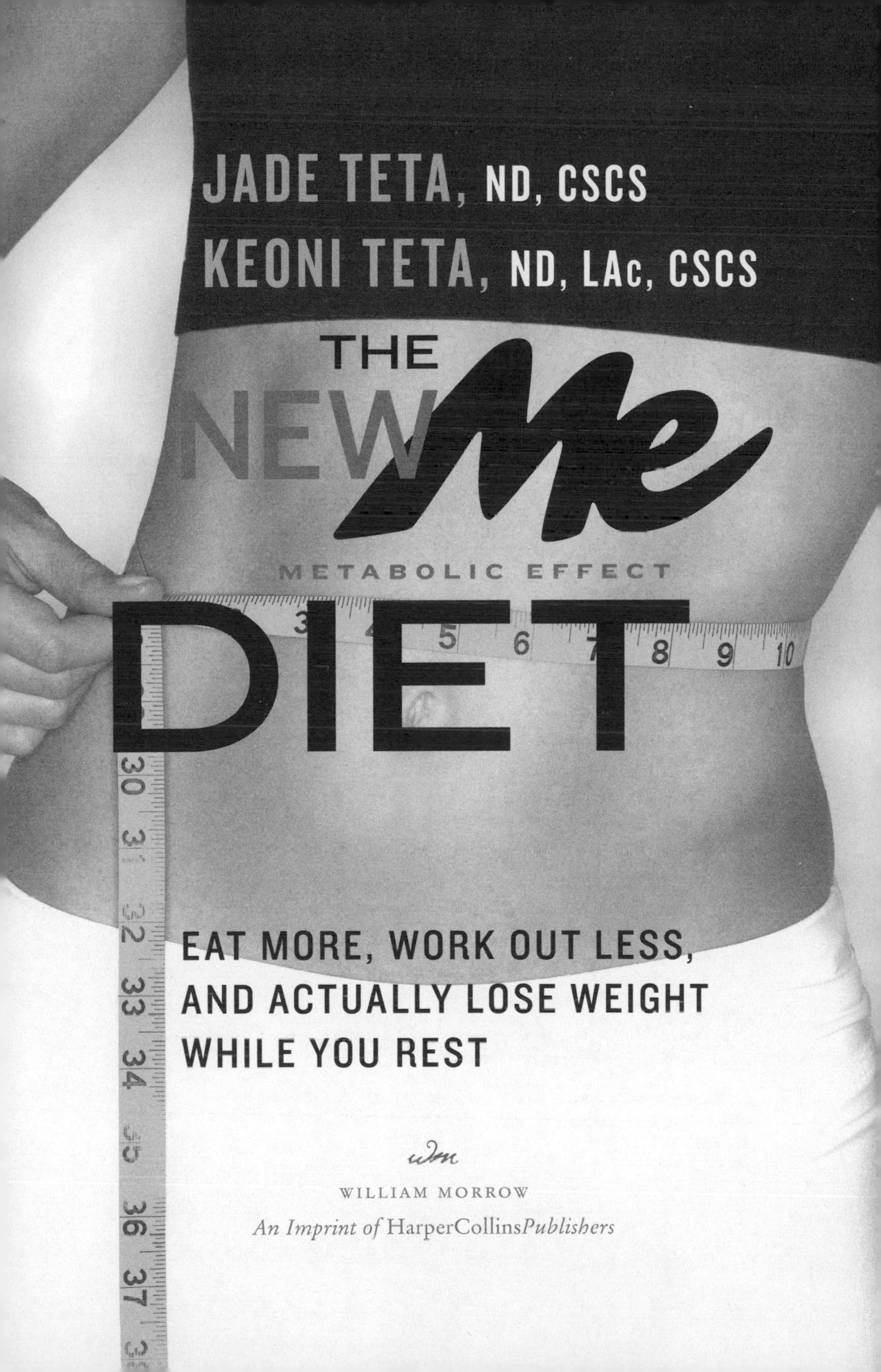

JADE TETA, ND, CSCS

KEONI TETA, ND, LAc, CSCS

THE NEW *Me*

METABOLIC EFFECT

DIET

EAT MORE, WORK OUT LESS,
AND ACTUALLY LOSE WEIGHT
WHILE YOU REST

WILLIAM MORROW

An Imprint of HarperCollinsPublishers

Metabolic Effect™, ME™, ME Fiber Complex™, ME Recovery Greens™, and ME Recovery Reds™ are registered trademarks.

All drawings are by John Stevens. All photographs are by Lisa Brewer. Image on page iii courtesy of Brand X Pictures/Jupiterimages.

HarperCollins books may be purchased for educational, business, or sales promotional use. For information please write: Special Markets Department, HarperCollins Publishers, 10 East 53rd Street, New York, NY 10022.

FIRST EDITION

Designed by Lisa Stokes
Title page designed by Richard L. Aquan

Library of Congress Cataloging-in-Publication Data

Teta, Jade.
   The new ME diet : eat more, work out less, and actually lose weight while you rest / Jade Teta and Keoni Teta. — 1st ed.
      p. cm.
  ISBN 978-0-06-183488-2
1. Weight loss. I. Teta, Keoni. II. Title.
  RM222.2.T4685 2009
  613.2'5—dc22

2009023458

10 11 12 13 14 OV/RRD 10 9 8 7 6 5 4 3 2 1

This book is dedicated to the dream that one day nutrition and exercise will replace pharmaceutical drugs as the cornerstone of a physician's education and will be used as the first line of defense for both the treatment and prevention of disease

CONTENTS

INTRODUCTION

Everyone knows how to get fit and lose weight: pedal your way through a 45-minute spinning class, spend 30 minutes like a hamster on the elliptical machine, or sprint on the treadmill 4 times a week. Oh, and go on a diet. Calories in. Calories out. Watch and weigh every morsel that goes in your mouth.

The problem with this low-calorie, aerobic-exercise model?

It doesn't work.

Are you shocked? Fitness experts have been telling us for decades that vigorous, one-size-fits-all aerobic exercise is the only way to reach optimal weight and muscle-to-fat ratio, i.e., to lose weight and look good.

The truth is that the typical aerobic-exercise program and calorie-counting diet burns muscle not fat. And fat is what you want to lose. In addition to making you look better, only fat loss has the power to restore a damaged metabolism and create lasting changes.

As holistic physicians, biochemists, and certified personal trainers, we know that the best way to get a lean, fit, and toned body lies with the ME Diet, a revolutionary approach to diet and exercise that requires just 30 minutes 3 times per week. Not only is the ME Diet supported by studies in physiology and fitness journals, but it has helped thousands of our clients accomplish weight loss and fitness goals beyond their dreams. How did this all come about?

Even though we're brothers and have been physically active since we were little boys, we've each had our own struggles with weight. In our Italian-American household, pasta was served at least 4 times a week, and our health-conscious mother rarely allowed us and our other siblings to have sweet cereals, soda, or fast food. A trip to McDonald's was a rare treat. Despite eating the same things when we were kids, we have very different body types. Jade tends to be heavier, while Keoni has always been thinner. Jade struggles to keep fat off his body; Keoni works to build muscle. Jade craves coffee and sweets; Keoni couldn't care less. Jade can drink five shots of espresso and sleep like a baby. If Keoni even smells a cup of coffee, he'll be awake for two days! On a cross-country driving trip, Keoni once drank a cup of coffee and was so wired that we had to pull over and let him run sprints. Despite sharing a similar genetic makeup and an identical diet growing up, we've always been aware of the differences between our metabolisms.

As we grew up and became interested in sports and fitness, we experimented with all kinds of diets. We tried "carbing up" before track meets. We drank 3,000-calorie protein shakes to gain weight for football. We researched and experimented with "performance-enhancing diets" and exercise programs. Some of our experiences seem comical when we look back at our efforts. We remember when Keoni was the fastest long-distance runner in the county during junior high school. Once at the county championships, Keoni scarfed down a large order of McDonald's french fries 30 minutes before a race. When the pistol fired, he took off and set a blistering pace but his legs began to shake during the last mile. He tried to push through until his legs became so heavy they just wouldn't cooperate. With the finish line in sight, Keoni seemed to be moving in slow motion, zigzagging all over the track with a look of horror on his face. As he weaved and wobbled, one racer after the next passed him. When he practically crawled over the finish line, our father looked at him in disbelief and said, "Jeez, son, what happened to you out there?" That was one of our first lessons in how food impacts performance.

Because of our fascination with nutrition and exercise, we became personal trainers in high school and developed dieting and fitness programs for our friends. We followed the standard thinking of the day—eat foods low in fat and high in carbs, and get plenty of aerobic exercise. It soon became obvious to us that this approach didn't work with most people. Even those who initially lost weight gained it all back and then some. At first, we assumed these people just weren't being compliant—they were not working out and were overeating. Like everyone else, we were taught that successful and permanent weight loss was simply a matter of genetics. Some people had either "fast" or "slow" metabolisms, and nothing could be done about it.

As with our research on performance nutrition, we studied and experimented with weight-loss programs as well. We tried every diet we knew of or heard about from our clients. We became vegetarians. Then we ate only raw foods. We tried low-fat and low-carb diets, calorie-counting programs, and juice fasts. But none of them worked when it came to permanent weight loss.

Going away to college and getting undergraduate degrees in biochemistry was the best thing that ever happened to us. Biochemistry, the study of chemistry in the human body, explains the reactions that occur within the body and how it uses food. Biochemistry taught us that the body does not act like a furnace, as the calorie-counting approach to food suggests. We learned that if you're lacking a certain vitamin or mineral, your metabolism slows down. If cell membranes are covered with the wrong types of fat, your metabolism falters. We found that if you eat sugar, your body releases hormones that make you store fat. With biochemistry we finally had an explanation for the differences in our bodies and a template for how the body really works.

We then observed how amateur and professional athletes trained, noting that the leanest athletes engaged in higher-intensity activity of shorter duration and ate more, not less, food. It was soon obvious that weight loss and fat loss are not the same—it is each person's individual biochemical reactions to exercise and food that drive fat burning or fat storage. In other words, just because someone burns calories or loses weight doesn't mean he or she is losing fat. We found that people who followed a low-calorie, high-aerobic program lost much needed muscle, rather than unnecessary body fat, which led to a less efficient metabolism in the long run.

When applying to medical school, we knew that our passion for fitness would become our profession, but we were shocked to learn that doctors receive absolutely no training in exercise and fitness, and almost no instruction in nutrition. We decided to attend Bastyr University, one of the few American medical schools specializing in holistic medicine, where nutrition and fitness are at the center of the program. After learning how the body reacts to hormone imbalances and uses a communication network to regulate its functions, we understood that hormones carry instructions to the cells, telling them how to behave and whether to release or hold on to fat stores. The types of calories are thus more important to hormones than the amount of calories, and certain compounds in food act like hormones themselves, interacting directly with human physiology and genes.

When we put this knowledge to work as personal trainers, we discovered that athletes train in a way that creates an optimal hormonal response in which the quality, not the quantity, of exercise and food is the driving factor in their success. Exercise and food carry information and instructions for the body, much like computer software. Some programs tell the body to store fat, while others signal it to burn fat. The messages sent depended on the individual nutritional makeup of each food or the specific type of exercise.

The more we used and tweaked these techniques, the more we saw our clients achieve consistent and sustained results. They lost inches, became more toned, built muscle mass, and looked more like athletes. They told us that they felt and functioned as if they were years younger.

Our greatest discovery was that each person is as different on the inside biochemically and hormonally as they are on the outside physically. While genetics play something of a role in our physiological makeup, choosing what we eat, how we exercise, and how we live has the most dramatic effect on our total well-being. The right foods, the right exercise, and the right lifestyle factors send signals that literally change the behavior of our bodies at the cellular and genetic levels, allowing each one of us to act almost as our own genetic engineers. By adjusting, modifying, and fine-tuning these parameters with tailored diet, exercise, and lifestyle inputs, we can have a tremendous impact on how we look and feel.

WHY THE METABOLIC EFFECT WORKS

So how does the program work? The ME Diet replaces the old science of calorie counting with the new science of hormonal fat burning. We know hormonal fat burning doesn't sound sexy, but it sure will make you look sexy. While eating less and exercising more may create a caloric deficit, your hormones unlock the fat-burning physiology—how cells, tissues, and organs function by themselves and with one another—that determines where those burned calories come from. Hormones not only predict the type of fuel a person will burn (sugar versus fat), but they also determine from where in the body that fuel will be taken (belly versus butt). The ME Diet combines the latest scientific research in endocrinology, exercise science, nutritional biochemistry, and strength and conditioning research, together with our years of experience and the results of thousands of satisfied clients to change your body's fat-burning physiology. Forever.

When most people think of hormones, reproductive steroids like estrogen, progesterone, and testosterone come to mind. The body, however, produces many hormones that have functions beyond reproduction. Hormones, or metabolic messengers, are chemicals, released by cells, that influence everything in the body, from stimulating or inhibiting growth to affecting moods. Certain hormones—insulin, cortisol, adrenaline, human growth hormone, and reproductive hormones—determine whether the body stores fat or burns it and where on the body fat is stored (perhaps the thighs or the arms), while indirectly controlling how hungry or full you feel. Leptin, ghrelin, and CCK are "hunger hormones" (although leptin also affects fat burning via its action on the thyroid gland), and others control the body's fat-burning physiology.

Well, then, shouldn't you be able to just "turn on" those hormones when you need them? Unfortunately, hormones lose their potency due to something called metabolic resistance. The effect is similar to walking into a room that has a strong smell. Upon entering the room, you are acutely aware of the smell and react to it by covering your nose and mouth. After some time, however, the smell becomes diminished or may not even be noticeable. When this happens to the metabolic messenger hormones, the body can no longer receive fat-burning signals. Metabolic resistance occurs when several hormones or just one key hormone (insulin, leptin, adrenaline) lose their fat-burning capabilities. The most common example is diabetes, in which insulin production is affected.

REBOOTING YOUR FAT-BURNING CAPABILITIES

The ME Diet reboots your damaged hormonal communication system and triggers its fat-burning capabilities. Sure, we could jump right into the nutritional information and workout routines, but the ME Diet is so revolutionary, so different from any other dietary-fitness program, it's important that you understand *how* it works.

In the first chapter we present the science behind why the ME Diet works and why so many programs you may have tried have not worked for you. These building blocks will give you the confidence to stick to the ME Diet and Workout so you can truly transform your body into the one you want.

In chapter two we help you figure out what type of burner you are. The ME Questionnaire gets to the heart of your eating habits and other lifestyle issues such as sleep, caffeine consumption, and reaction to bright lights (these factors also play an important role as hormonal stimulators) to determine whether you are a muscle burner, sugar burner, or mixed burner. If you're a sugar burner, for instance, then you should reduce the amount of starchy foods, focus on plenty of protein, eat more vegetables than fruit, and stick with less-sweet fruits like apples, berries, and pears. A mixed burner or a muscle burner can tolerate higher amounts of starchy foods and has more options for fruits and vegetables according to specific lists. (Why the differences? The hormonal response to starch is more dramatic in sugar burners, while higher amounts of starch are less detrimental to mixed burners and can actually benefit muscle burners. By eliminating certain fruits from their diets, sugar burners can rev up their fat-burning mechanisms. Mixed burners, on the other hand, have a more balanced physiology and most fruit sugars don't slow their machinery as dramatically.)

You'll then learn how to fuel your body with the appropriate foods and will discover a new way of eating that will activate those important fat-burning hormones. The ME Diet replaces the calorie-counting model with bite counting and weekly Reward Meals (which help you exert control over your body's hunger thermostat), and a food plan tailored to your body's specific burner type.

The next step is a unique, high-intensity exercise program that combines weight training and cardiovascular routines with critical rest periods in one 30-minute workout. Very specific hybrid exercises are used to generate a cardiovascular stimulus in addition to a resistance-training effect; together the resistance and cardiovascular response trigger the specific hormones (metabolic messengers) that burn fat, not muscle. In other words, the two work synergistically. They also create an afterburn that benefits the body long after the workout is over and amplifies the fat-burning effects of low-intensity activities like walking. Your body will become firm and toned, with the trim silhouette you've always wanted. Gone are the flabby arms, saggy thighs, and jiggling love handles you thought you were stuck with.

Coupling this practical diet and exercise program with lifestyle adjustments in sleep patterns, alcohol and coffee consumption, and stress level, you will experience the ME Diet in three stages: the Metabolic Spark, the Metabolic Transformation, and the Metabolic Effect. In the first 3 weeks to 3 months, you'll jump-start your stalled metabolism and lose 5 to 15 pounds of water weight, which signals that your metabolism is ready to begin burning fat. When this Metabolic Spark occurs, you'll begin experiencing a Metabolic Transformation, losing 0.5 to 2 percent of body fat a week, until you reach optimal metabolic functioning: the Metabolic Effect. Don't believe us? Just ask one of the ten thousand people who have seen results from our program!

CHAPTER ONE

HOW THE ME DIET WORKS

Think about the differences between elite sprinters and marathoners. Both are extremely lean, but sprinters look muscular and trim while long-distance runners look gaunt and thin. Sprinters engage in very short bursts of all-out effort for seconds or, at most, minutes. They burn far fewer calories when training for and engaging in their sport. And they have less body fat and higher amounts of muscle mass. Surprisingly, marathoners, who run for hours, have more body fat and expend much larger amounts of caloric energy. Shouldn't this make marathoners leaner than sprinters? If the aerobic-exercise and calorie-cutting model was the final word on fat loss, there wouldn't be such a discrepancy between these two types of athletes. And if elite marathoners have a greater percentage of body fat and less muscle mass, then how can the traditional diet and aerobic-exercise program be expected to work for the average person?

Similarly, some people are in good shape and exercise at the gym 3 or 4 times a week, working up a sweat and getting their heart rates to their proper levels with no problem. But what happens when they climb two flights of stairs and they're suddenly breathless and their legs are burning by the time they reach the top? They think, "What's wrong with me? I work out all the time!" Why can they feel fine after a workout, but winded after climbing two flights of stairs? The answer is because virtually every popular commercial program, fad diet, or exercise protocol in the world is currently concerned with any old type of weight loss and does nothing to change your body to lose the right weight and work better.

The above contradictions are easily explained by understanding how hormones are able to manipulate fat burning. Hormones in this book refer to all signaling molecules (i.e., hormones, neurotransmitters, and others). Think of the body as an engine that can choose between two fuels—fat and sugar. The body can also use protein as a fuel, but it is converted to sugar before it can be burned. This means muscle tissue can be a significant source of sugar energy in certain people. Fat is analogous to diesel fuel; it will drive your body for long distances, but it doesn't provide much in the way of performance. High-octane sugar delivers exceptional performance, but dreadful mileage. How you exercise and what you eat determines which hormonal messengers are triggered to burn fat or sugar.

When these fat-burning hormones are activated, the response is what we call the Metabolic Effect, an optimal state of hormonal balance that enhances utilization of the body's fat stores. Changing specific lifestyle choices like exercise and diet are the chief means of accessing this highly beneficial state. This is why the ME diet is so different. Where other programs focus on the *quantity* of food eaten or the amount of exercise done, the ME diet focuses on the *quality* of these inputs. Exercise and food are information for the body, and the quality of that information determines the metabolic outcome.

Muscle Loss Versus Fat Loss: What's the Difference?

Muscle loss is disastrous for your metabolism; the ability to burn fat becomes drastically reduced without it.

Grab the thigh or the back of someone's arm. A complete lack of tone and saggy skin is a dead giveaway that she or he has been a serial dieter. Because traditional exercise and weight-loss regimens don't discriminate between the types of tissue, muscle is usually lost just as readily as fat.

Muscle tissue can inherently change its shape with exercise and diet. Fat tissue can't do this. When muscle tissue is increased with the ME Diet, the connective tissue is strengthened and pulls the skin tighter. Fat tissue, on the other hand, makes you bigger as you gain fat and smaller when you lose it, but fat cannot produce contour, shape, and tone. During the Metabolic Spark, you will begin to see and feel contours in your body that are impossible to achieve with low-calorie and aerobic-dominated programs. If you have lost a lot of muscle mass, this stage may take three months so that additional muscle can be added to your frame through exercise and diet.

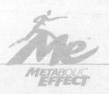

WHY TRADITIONAL EXERCISE REGIMENS AND DIETS DON'T WORK

Every day men and women of all ages come to us with the same stories: after diligently following programs that have promised to keep them thin, fit, and healthy, they haven't lost weight or changed the look of their bodies. The truth is that calorie-counting diets and exhausting exercise routines just don't work in the long run. People who embark on calorie-burning and aerobic weight-loss programs face an uphill struggle. Most last only a few days. Even those who are able to stick with such a program find it a constant battle just to maintain their hard-won results.

Even the research studies on the best weight-loss programs boast a short-term success rate of only 20 percent (short-term success is defined as achieving and maintaining weight loss for over 1 year). That means 80 percent of those who try these programs have no success at all or fail to maintain their weight loss for more than 1 year!

In other words, if you went on a calorie-restricted diet and aerobic-exercise program every year for five years straight, you would fail every year except for one. Your chances of success are much less than 50 percent. With odds like that, why not just flip a coin and eat whatever you like and give up all exercise? Many people do.

It gets worse. The success rate of achieving and maintaining weight loss for more than two years is often cited as 5 percent. So even if you did make it through the first year just fine, you are even less likely to have continued success in the second year. The worst of it is the way experts define success. A reduction in weight of 5 to 10 percent maintained for a year is considered a success according to most experts. For one of our clients, a 160-pound woman, this amounts to an average weight loss of about 12 pounds over 12 months. She struggled for 3 months and lost 5 pounds on a low-calorie diet before coming to us. If she was able to maintain the program for another 9 months, she might have lost another 7 pounds. At the end of a year, would she have been any happier with the result? Furthermore, would the weight she lost have been mostly muscle or fat? While a 10 percent loss in body weight has health benefits, it is far from the transformation most people seek. Not to mention that all these numbers actually mean very little in real-world terms because popular weight-loss programs never measure what type of weight was lost. And it is fat we want to lose and muscle we want to keep.

The most tragic thing about all these diet stories and studies is that the same scenarios are being played out everywhere. The same people who fail at these programs are the ones who attempt the identical thing 3 to 6 months down the line. This is why it's called yo-yo dieting.

Hormones Versus Calories

There's an ongoing debate between exercise and nutrition experts about the hormonal effects of food versus counting calories. The truth is that both matter. In order to lose weight you must have a caloric deficit, but to burn fat you need a caloric deficit *and* metabolic hormones must be in balance. A doughnut and a chicken breast may have the same number of calories and you'll lose weight if you eat less of them, but each one sends different messages to the body. The chicken breast will send signals that give you a better sense of well-being and enable your physiology to function well. Your metabolic messenger hormones like leptin and ghrelin control hunger; neurohormones like serotonin, dopamine, and GABA impact motivation, focus, and well-being; insulin, cortisol, glucagon, human growth hormone, and testosterone all impact fat and muscle storage or breakdown. If you can balance your hormones, you will eat less without even being consciously aware of it and the calories will take care of themselves. This is the key difference between weight loss and fat loss.

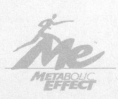

THE HORMONES THAT TRIGGER THE METABOLIC EFFECT

The ME Diet focuses on the nine hormones that are critical to fat burning and getting your body on the right track:

Adrenaline is the gas-pedal hormone. When the ME Diet program is used, adrenaline signals the body to begin burning fuel. A chain reaction then causes the release of other hormones—cortisol, testosterone, and HGH—to be triggered and the body goes into a fat-burning mode. When adrenaline is released in someone with high insulin and leptin levels, the body switches to a sugar-burning mode. The ME nutrition and exercise program releases the proper hormonal balance and gets the body burning *fat*.

Cortisol is the Jekyll-and-Hyde hormone. It can be your best friend or worst enemy when it comes to fat burning. Cortisol released in the presence of high insulin levels, low testosterone, and limited HGH (human growth hormone) acts as an unfriendly fat-storing and muscle-burning hormone. If cortisol is released with large amounts of HGH and testosterone, it becomes a good friend, blocking muscle burning while enhancing the fat-burning effect.

Ghrelin is called the stomach-growl hormone. Even its pronunciation sounds like a growl. Ghrelin affects hunger from hour to hour, while leptin affects it from day to day. As ghrelin levels rise, hunger signals are sent to the brain. High ghrelin levels are very difficult to overcome through willpower alone. Eating protein and fiber and doing intense exercise can blunt ghrelin's message.

Glucagon is insulin's alter ego. If insulin makes you store fat, then glucagon helps burn it. Glucagon works in the liver to help it regulate both sugar and fat usage. The insulin/glucagon ratio is a major determinant of whether you burn or store fat. In general, starches/sugar secrete insulin, while protein stimulates glucagon, so adjusting the protein/carb balance favors fat burning.

Insulin is a storing and locking hormone. When it comes to storing fat, high insulin levels assure that any extra calories be stored as fat, while putting a lock on fat cells and inhibiting the body's ability to release fat. Carbohydrates (starches, sweets, processed foods) impact dramatically on elevating insulin levels, increasing fat storage and decreasing fat burning.

Leptin is the body's fuel gauge. It controls how hungry you are on a day-to-day basis. If you become leptin resistant, you will eat and eat and eat as if you are starving. This is why some people become morbidly obese; their bodies never receive the message to stop eating and start burning. The ME Diet program reactivates the body's response to leptin.

Testosterone and HGH (human growth hormone) are the building and burning hormones. They send signals to be lean and muscular, and work with cortisol and adrenaline to assure that fat is burned rather than stored.

The *thyroid* stabilizes metabolism and takes its cues from other hormones (like leptin) to maintain weight set point; it acts like a weight thermostat. Many people with underactive thyroid function are actually suffering from a deficit in leptin signaling because their bodies are leptin resistant. Leptin acts on the thyroid by stimulating the release of its fat-burning hormones.

Metabolism from the Hormonal Perspective

The FAT "Storer"		The FAT "Burner"	
HORMONE LEVELS		HORMONE LEVELS	
Glucagon	Low ▼	Glucagon	High ▲
Cortisol	High ▲	Cortisol	Low ▼
Human Growth Hormone	Low ▼	Human Growth Hormone	High ▲
Insulin	High ▲	Insulin	Low ▼
Leptin	High ▲	Leptin	Low ▼

HORMONES ARE LIKE PEOPLE

You've been invited to a formal gathering of your professional peers. Chances are that you'll dress less casually than usual (no jeans or T-shirts). You'll be more reserved and polite and engage in appropriate conversation. If going out for drinks with a group of close friends, it's likely that you'll dress less formally, speak louder, and laugh more. Conversation will be relaxed and you'll feel more comfortable, less uptight. In other words, the way you behave depends on the situation.

Hormones work in the same way. Whether you burn fat or store fat has everything to do with the interactions of hormones. Cortisol, often seen as a fat-storing hormone, actually either enhances fat usage or stimulates fat storage depending on other hormone ratios. Cortisol, along with human growth hormone and testosterone, is a magical combination elicited by the ME Workouts and is partially responsible for the enhanced afterburn of these workouts.

When cortisol and insulin get together, they're a particularly troublesome pair. If you eat sugar or a large amount of food, insulin is released. Because the body can use only a small amount of sugar at one time, the amount of sugar in a plate of pasta will send insulin to very high levels because insulin can push sugar out of the blood and into the cells for storage as sugar or fat. This insulin surge causes blood sugar levels to lower undesirably very quickly. To keep blood sugar levels stable, cortisol will be released to raise blood sugar.

Depending on how well tuned your metabolism is, this back-and-forth game of insulin and cortisol can go on and on all day, causing mood swings, energy lows, and metabolic resistance that leads to fat storage, especially around the middle of the body. This is one of the most insidious hormonal effects of our modern lifestyle, as this seesawing can be triggered by stress or high starch/sugar foods and ultimately leads to obesity, diabetes, and other medical issues.

YOUR METABOLIC ORGANS

The inability to turn on fat burning is often related to the organs and tissues responsible for making, releasing, or reacting to your metabolic messengers. The adrenal glands, the pancreas, the liver, and muscle and fat tissues are the most important ones.

Adrenal Glands

These can best be described as your body's alarm system because they secrete the major stress hormones adrenaline, noradrenaline, and cortisol. Not only do these hormones wake us up in the morning, but they also help regulate blood sugar, heart rate, and moods. The body's ability to burn fat is directly related to the adrenal hormone reserves. Chronic stress and poor eating habits force the adrenal glands to work overtime, resulting in tiredness, lack of motivation, and joint and muscle pain. Muscle burners are especially susceptible to this because their adrenal glands are constantly running in overdrive.

Fat

Fat is a type of body tissue and a hormone-secreting organ. Fat tissue releases many powerful hormones, including leptin, inflammatory compounds, and even estrogen and cortisol. Fat deposits act differently depending on where they are on the body. For instance, belly fat secretes more detrimental hormones than deposits on thighs. Sugar burners especially have issues with the release of fat-storing hormones from fat and tend to produce greater amounts of leptin, inflammatory molecules, estrogen, and cortisol from fat cells, which together create a negative fat-storing effect.

Pancreas

This organ releases insulin and glucagon in response to food and to stress. Sugar burners often have an exaggerated insulin response to foods in the same way muscle burners have an overactive adrenal response. Over time, this leads to insulin resistance, obesity, diabetes, and possibly pancreatic failure. Sugar burners must be extra careful to limit sugary foods and overeating to keep the pancreas healthy. The relative strengths or weaknesses of the pancreas and adrenal glands are the major difference between sugar burners and muscle burners.

Liver

The liver is the body's major detoxification center and a primary site of hormone action. Stress, environmental toxins, and especially high-fat and high-sugar diets wreak havoc on the liver, which may result in high cholesterol and triglycerides and elevated liver enzymes. Sugar burners are often the most susceptible to liver problems.

Muscle

Muscle is technically tissue, but we include it with other metabolic organs because it consumes most of the body's energy. While muscle is important for movement, it's also a major hub of hormonal activity and a major source of metabolic messengers. When muscle mass is lost due to lack of exercise, poor nutrition, and stress, it negatively impacts the metabolism as a whole. Mixed burners often have balanced responses in adrenal, liver, and pancreas function. Their issues come from muscle loss due to a sedentary lifestyle, which can give rise to problems in other organ tissues. Restoring lost muscle is the first step for many mixed burners.

OKAY, I UNDERSTAND THAT CERTAIN HORMONES CAN BURN FAT, BUT WHAT IS THE ME DIET?

Specific metabolic messengers—hormones—are stimulated through a high-protein/high-fiber/modified-carb diet that is individualized depending on your burner type. This diet works in concert with a rest-based, hybrid weight-training workout done at an individual's fitness level. Every time we eat or exercise we have the opportunity to turn on or off a fat-calorie afterburn, which we call the Metabolic Effect. But with the ME Diet, the difference lies in the quality of the exercise or diet, not the quantity. Diet and exercise work synergistically, triggering peak hormonal and muscle responses. With 6 meals a day and 30 minutes of exercise 3 times per week, along with walking, these metabolic messengers stimulate the body to build muscle and burn fat quickly and efficiently.

WHY IS THE ME DIET BETTER THAN THE TRADITIONAL AEROBIC-EXERCISE MODEL?

The ME Diet includes a fitness program designed to work with the body to trigger fat-burning hormones and keep you lean, toned, and fit. It is the way humans were designed to move and the way athletes exercise. What is most remarkable is that this fat-burning mechanism continues for 16 to 48 hours once the actual workout is over!

Ninety percent of all sports combine elements of aerobic exercise and resistance training/anaerobic exercise, yet almost every popular exercise program separates the two. The ME Diet offers a workout regimen that efficiently burns fat, resulting in significant weight loss and a lean, toned body.

WHY AEROBIC EXERCISE DOESN'T BURN FAT:
EPOC—EXCESS POSTEXERCISE OXYGEN CONSUMPTION

While the ME Workout modulates hormones so more fat and calories can be burned during activity, the program also creates a metabolic "ripple" effect of enhanced fat burning that lasts for hours and even days after a workout is over. This increased energy use after a workout is referred to as excess postexercise oxygen consumption, or EPOC. EPOC, also called oxygen debt, measures how much oxygen the body consumes in the hours and days after a workout and is the scientific name for what we call the Metabolic Effect.

For an example of EPOC, or oxygen debt, think about what happens after climbing several flights of stairs. While walking up the stairs, breathing is labored, but respiration becomes most difficult once the top is reached. The body does this to recover the "debt" of oxygen created during the intense activity. This is just a miniexample of the much larger metabolic effect produced by proper hormonal exercise. The amount of oxygen consumed is directly correlated to how much energy is burned, but it is hormones that determine whether that energy is mostly fat or sugar. Low-intensity aerobic-driven exercise, such as jogging, swimming, and bike riding, does not produce an adequate EPOC effect and is an inferior fat-burning strategy.

While hormonal influences on fat burning are a novel concept to some, it is a far more powerful model than caloric metabolism. Here's how it works: Exercise of sufficient intensity elevates stress hormones like adrenaline, noradrenaline, and cortisol. This creates a chain reaction, which, with intense exercise, leads to the buildup of lactic acid. This is where the magic of the metabolic effect kicks in.

Lactic acid is often seen as a metabolic waste product, but

it is the physiological biofeedback/signaling molecule that triggers the release of two of the most powerful fat-burning hormones: testosterone and HGH (human growth hormone). The entire "hormonal soup" (adrenaline, noradrenaline, and cortisol, with testosterone and HGH) is what drives the EPOC effect. These hormones are the key to the ME Diet because their combined action is responsible for the caloric afterburn created by EPOC, and they ensure that the calories that are burned come from fat. The key metabolic messengers that begin the EPOC effect, adrenaline and noradrenaline, cause the body to switch to high-octane sugar usage, which historically supplied humans with the energy to survive life-threatening events. This chemical release (the adrenaline/noradrenaline effect, aka the fight-or-flight response) was always followed by a burst of intense movement to capture food or avoid danger, which is why low-intensity activity (i.e., aerobic exercise) does not create the metabolic effect. Only high-intensity exercise creates the hormonal burst to create the EPOC effect that science has shown can last up to 48 hours after the workout.

The major failure of calorie-driven aerobic exercise is that it does not impact these hormones in the same way and therefore is unable to trigger the metabolic effect. Aerobic activity by its very nature never reaches a high enough intensity to turn on the adrenaline response necessary to trigger EPOC and the metabolic effect. This is the reason sprinters have less fat and are more muscular than marathon runners.

WHO CAN BENEFIT FROM THE ME DIET?

Everyone. The brilliance of the ME diet is that it can be individually geared to and maintained by people of all different metabolisms, fitness levels, and lifestyles—from beginners to triathletes, from young people to seniors. Each person eats according to the way his or her body works and exercises to generate the precise amount of intensity necessary to trigger the metabolic effect required. The result is a lean, toned body with a smaller body-fat percentage.

WHAT KIND OF EQUIPMENT IS NECESSARY?

A pair of dumbbells. That's it. Choose a free weight that allows you to do 3 perfect bicep curls, not 2, not 4, but 3. Then divide the number of pounds in that weight by half. That is the amount of weight you will use for the workout. So, if you can do 3 perfect bicep curls with 20-pound weights, then use 10-pound weights for your workout. This quick, efficient method gives you an appropriate starting weight to begin with. Some people will start with 2-pound weights; others will require 12 or 20 pounds. The amount of weight used will increase based on your performance during the workout.

WHAT IS THE ME DIET WORKOUT?

There are 4 groups of hybrid exercises with 4 exercises in each group, all of which are explained and illustrated. Choose one exercise from each group for a total of 4 exercises per workout. Do 12 reps of each of the four exercises in circuit fashion. As you perform each exercise, you will need to rest, because the muscles are burning and/or the lungs are working too hard *or* the weight is too heavy to lift. At this point, rest for as long as necessary. Then continue exactly where you left off. You will circuit through the 4 exercises back-to-back for 20 minutes, attempting to complete as many rounds as possible with the goal of doing 5 rounds. If you can complete more than 5 rounds, you need to increase the weight by 2.5 to 5 pounds in each hand at your next workout. Choose a new workout as often as you like, but we recommend staying with the same one for a minimum of 6, but no more than 12 workouts.

THE ME WORKOUT

Rest-Based Training allows each person to generate the correct intensity necessary to turn on fat burning long after the workout is over. The push-until-you-have-to-rest format allows participants to benefit from the latest fat-burning research. Hybrid exercises combine upper and lower body movements and simultaneously tax the aerobic and anaerobic systems. The ME Workout uses these exercises exclusively because they have been shown to almost double the amount of calories burned in a workout. More important, the massive amount of muscle recruited is able to generate an intense burst of hormonal activity that creates the desired EPOC afterburn. In volumes 94 (2005) and 97 (2006) of the *European Journal of Physiology,* two studies showed that combined lower and upper body workouts were able to improve muscle mass, lower body fat, and improve multiple fitness parameters in as little as 8 weeks. Thigh and abdominal fat measured in the second study decreased by 11 percent and 12 percent respectively in a 14-week period, while the muscle cross-sectional area increased between 2 percent and 14 percent in 9 out of 10 muscles measured.

HOW DO I KNOW IF I'M DOING THE ME WORKOUT PROPERLY?

The ME Workout uses a 1 to 4 rating scale, called the Metabolic Exertion Scale, to determine how people at any fitness level can use the workout and tailor it to their individual abilities.

1. You are at rest and are not exerting yourself.

2. Exercise is easy. You can still talk. You feel no burn in your muscles and/or the weight feels easy to lift.

3. You are working out hard. You are no longer able to talk. Your muscles are burning and/or the weight is very heavy. You are starting to generate a metabolic effect!

4. You can no longer continue to exercise. You experience severe muscle burn and/or the weight feels too heavy. You have to rest. At this point, the metabolic effect is drastically enhanced, with an increase in the muscle-building, fat-burning hormones. This number 4 stage is what we call the Metabolic Effect Point. Go back to number 1 and start again.

DO I HAVE TO "REST"?

Absolutely! The rest stage is required because without it you will automatically pace yourself (aerobic exercise) and not breach the intensity threshold needed to release the growth-promoting, fat-burning hormones. This is what we call Rest-Based Training (RBT), and is a concept unique to the ME system. This workout is effective because of the burst of hormones it creates (HGH, testosterone, adrenaline, etc.). The problem is that aerobic exercise by its very definition needs to be below a certain intensity, because once you go over that intensity you are anaerobic or superaerobic. As soon as you cross into anaerobic metabolism, the body reacts by generating large amounts of hormones responsible for the afterburn, or the metabolic effect. You cannot reach this state aerobically because the intensity threshold (i.e., the anaerobic state) is never achieved. The more you rest, the harder you will push. The harder you push, the more you have to rest. And the better results you will achieve.

PACING VERSUS PUSHING: REST-BASED TRAINING

Interval training, alternating periods of hard exercise with periods of easy exercise, takes advantage of rest periods inserted into the workout and has been shown to reliably stimulate EPOC. Rest-based workouts differ from interval training because there is no set time limit on how long to work and when to rest. Interval training prescribes a very definitive "work phase" with a finite "rest phase," which, like aerobic exercise, may lead to "pacing yourself." Rest-Based Training eliminates the pacing effect by "pushing yourself" until you can no longer perform the exercises, then resting until you can begin again. The mantra to remember is "Push until you can't and rest until you can." It's this Rest-Based Training approach that allows exercisers of all fitness levels to generate the exact intensity necessary to experience the metabolic afterburn/EPOC.

Elite athletes cannot sustain an all-out effort for more than 60 seconds, which means the average exerciser's full-speed limitations are probably closer to 15 to 30 seconds. Some interval routines prescribe intervals of up to 4 minutes in length, which means that pacing will still occur. Pacing is the antithesis of intensity and is the very reason aerobic exercise fails to adequately burn fat.

While interval training is definitely superior to standard aerobic exercise in terms of generating results, the Rest-Based Training in the ME Workout takes it one step further. In rest-based workouts, the goal is to push as hard as possible for as long as possible with no pacing whatsoever. When you can't perform even one more exercise because your muscles are so exhausted, you rest just until you have recovered enough—a matter of seconds to minutes—to start the exercise again and deliver the same degree of intensity. This means that anyone at any fitness level can self-tailor the workout to his or her exact specifications. An elite athlete may be able to go all out for a minute in a full-throttle sprint, while an older adult may be able to last only 10 seconds in a fast-paced walk. The ME Workout allows people at all fitness levels to benefit from the metabolic afterburn created from intense exercise.

HOW MANY TIMES A WEEK SHOULD I DO THE ME WORKOUT?

Just 3 times a week. Devote 20 minutes to the core exercises in the ME Workout. On all days, especially those when you're not doing the hybrid exercises, walk for 30 to 60 minutes. Think of a walk as a necessity, not exercise. Our human ancestors walked all day, every day! When walking is combined with the high-intensity weight exercises, the two work synergistically to enhance fat burning.

YOUR ANCESTRAL METABOLISM

Whether or not you realize it, you are the genetic equal of cavemen. Although each one of us is unique, we all share the same basic metabolic tendencies of our hunter-gatherer ancestors. Humans evolved for millions of years on this planet in an environment that shaped our species. To get an idea of what life was like, imagine you lived in a neighborhood without grocery stores, convenience stores, fast-food restaurants, or Starbucks. Imagine that all you had were the wild animals running around in the woods and the wild plant life around you. Your food supply consisted of wild animals you caught and vegetables and fruits that grew nearby. You walked all day every day gathering food, finding shelter, fetching water, and doing other tasks for survival. You fought off predators. You hauled, lifted, and climbed. When the sun went down you slept. This is what your metabolism and your body are designed for—eating lean animal protein and vegetables and fruits, being active, and getting a good night's sleep.

HOW SOON WILL I SEE RESULTS FROM THE ME DIET?

Immediately. First, your new eating pattern will raise your energy levels, reduce hunger, and balance food cravings. With the ME Workout, there's a combined sense of feeling energized and exhilarated as well as spent and fatigued. In a matter of 2 to 3 weeks, you will notice that your face is thinner, your body is more toned, and there's a weight loss of 5 to 15 pounds! You will continue to see a steady drop in body fat as you continue the ME Diet. The specific diet and rest-based workouts work to enhance each other and are inseparable. If you just do the exercises without changing your eating habits, or vice versa, the results will be modest, if there are any at all.

Marcus: Working Out to Lose Fat

Marcus, now 36 years old, was a jock in high school and played basketball on his school's team. When he hit 30 it seemed like he started to put on weight overnight. By 34, he was obese, weighing 260 pounds with 32 percent body fat. He went on a low-carb diet and exercised for 2 hours a day, 6 days a week. It took him about 4 months to lose 30 pounds and his body fat dropped to 26 percent.

Despite weighing less, his body shape hadn't changed much; he was still carrying fat around his middle. No matter what he did—spinning classes, jogging, biking—he couldn't lose that rubber tire. He was always hungry and constantly craved sweets.

Like many people who become gym addicts, Marcus soon discovered that he couldn't spend 2 hours every day in the gym, and he went back to his old eating habits. In the next 2 months his weight quickly ballooned back up to 260 pounds, with 35 percent body fat.

Since Marcus could no longer devote all that time to working out, he was intrigued by the ME classes at his gym. Instead of spinning away on a bike, like a hamster, he started working out three days a week doing 30-minute ME classes, followed by 30 minutes of rest-based intervals. He went from 12 hours each week to just 3!

He immediately began to see changes in his body, but his weight remained the same when he stepped on the scale. How was that possible? Because he was losing inches—body fat—which he measured on his handheld body fat machine.

Marcus was a mixed burner, so instead of cutting out all carbs, he ate more protein and controlled his carbs by having just ten bites of them at each meal. As a result, the insulin in his body helped him build muscle. In the next 9 months, Marcus lost 40 pounds and went from 35 percent body fat to 19 percent body fat. His waist size went from 42 inches to 36 inches.

Marcus still works out 30 minutes 3 times a week and has become a certified ME trainer and one of our most talented instructors.

DO I HAVE TO CHANGE THE WAY I EAT?

Yes. The two biggest influences on your fat-burning machinery are food and exercise. But don't worry. Because the exercise and diet work with the body's innate intelligence, you will naturally feel more satisfied and unconsciously choose foods that support the metabolic effect. Like exercise, food releases powerful metabolic messengers every time you eat something. What these messengers say depends on what you eat. Every time you eat you have the opportunity to send the signal for fat burning or fat storage. We explain throughout what to eat to get the best results with the ME Diet.

WHAT TO EAT FOR THE ME DIET

We don't believe in counting calories. Yes, you read that correctly. With the ME Diet what kind of foods you eat is more important than how much you eat. Hunger, cravings, and energy levels are the body's biofeedback tools. By adjusting dietary approaches based on these hormonally controlled sensations, the ME program adjusts perfectly to the individual. Certain high-protein and -fiber foods—such as chicken breasts and broccoli—can be eaten in large quantities, yet still turn on the body's fat-burning mechanism because of the specific metabolic messengers they stimulate. This stimulation leads to a unique hormonal response characterized by decreased ghrelin, increased glucagon, balanced leptin, improved dopamine signaling, and stimulated growth hormones. Together these lead to a fat-burning and muscle-building effect that can last for several hours after the meal. The best part is that this hormonal effect decreases hunger sensations, improves energy, and makes cravings disappear. When the body is appropriately fed, it responds with optimal function. The ideal metabolic effect.

Like exercise, the quality—or type—of food consumed matters more than the quantity. The relative macronutrient composition of a meal determines the hormonal influence on fuel metabolism. Protein consumption increases glucagon relative to insulin, while carbohydrates do the reverse. This unique hormonal balance enhances fat usage and what is known as the thermic effect of food, which is an increased period of calorie usage induced by foods with extra protein and fiber that stimulate enhanced fat burning. In this way, the metabolic effect is created by food and can last for several hours after eating. Fat is hormonally neutral in most cases, but its effects can be altered by carbohydrates. Together, carbohydrates and fat have a detrimental effect on fat burning because they elevate the fat-storing hormones more than either one would individually. By increasing the percentage of protein and fiber in the diet, the ME Diet program elevates glucagon while lowering insulin and increasing fat burning. While many hormone-savvy experts argue about the proper ratio of carbohydrates to protein, the ME program recognizes that everyone is different and uses an approach that teaches people to tailor their diets to their individual food needs.

Our clients tell us that they don't have the time to spend on shopping for and preparing elaborate meals, so all of our food suggestions for meals and snacks are created for busy people on the go. Smoothies with protein powder and frozen fruit can be blended in seconds. Pick up a roast chicken on the way home from work. Keep cut-up fruits and vegetables in the fridge and protein bars on hand so there's always something healthy to nip those hunger pangs before they take over! Throughout the book, we offer lots of tips and ideas for making healthy food choices.

Human metabolism is intelligent and ordered. On the one hand, we're all uniquely different from one another, while on the other, we all share the same basic physiological processes that were honed during evolution. It's important to look at food and exercise as information that you can use as an individual. Remember, every time you eat and exercise you have the ability to send a fat-burning message to your body.

CHAPTER TWO

WHAT KIND OF BURNER ARE YOU?

As far as your body is concerned, it's either storing fat or burning it. Your body doesn't care about how much you weigh. Your weight is misleading in helping you determine if you are a fat burner or not. Your metabolism, on the other hand, is determined by the unique interaction of your body's individual biochemistry and your environment. By environment, we mean your lifestyle choices—what you eat and drink, how much (or how little) exercise and sleep you get, how much stress you are under, what chemicals and toxins you are exposed to, and every other conceivable interaction with the world around you.

The body has three fuels—protein (muscle), sugar, and fat—at its disposal for burning. When protein is burned, it becomes sugar, making us all either sugar or fat burners. We burn both fuels all the time, but individual metabolic tendencies make some of us burn more sugar and others burn more fat. The goal of the ME Diet is to make your body burn fat efficiently.

When someone comes to our center, we perform sophisticated metabolic and genetic testing on blood samples to determine the specific fitness plan and diet needed to switch the body's metabolism and get results. We realize that's not possible for everyone, so we've streamlined our scientific procedure into this simple questionnaire to determine whether you are a sugar burner, a muscle burner, or a mixed burner.

THE METABOLIC EFFECT QUESTIONNAIRE

To find out what kind of fuel burner you are—sugar, muscle, or mixed—answer each question to the best of your ability. Don't stop and think about the details, just circle the answer that fits you the best. If none of the answers suits you, then choose the one that is closest.

1. Which of the following meals would give you sustained and lasting energy if it were the only meal you could eat all day?

    a. Cereal (0)
    b. Eggs and cereal (+1)
    c. Steak and eggs (+2)

2. What best describes your reaction to high-carbohydrate foods such as pasta or potatoes?

    a. They give me a short boost in energy, but I can crash later. (+1)
    b. They make me feel tired and lethargic almost immediately after eating them. (+2)
    c. They give me long-lasting energy. (-2)

3. When it comes to desserts, which do you prefer?

    a. I have no preference. (+1)
    b. Creamy, rich sweets like cheesecake or chocolate mousse. (+2)

    c. I like all sweets, but prefer lighter things like cookies and candy bars. (0)

4. What best describes your reaction to eating protein such as chicken, steak, or eggs?

    a. They satisfy my hunger and give me energy for many hours. (+4)

    b. They give me about the same energy as carbohydrate-rich foods such as pasta and potatoes. (+1)

    c. They fill me up and often make me feel sluggish and tired *or* I do not eat meat. (-2)

5. Which do you crave the most?

    a. Protein, salt, and coffee. (+2)

    b. Sugar; coffee; or cocktails, wine, or beer. (-2)

    c. I don't get cravings very often, but when I do, I crave a. and b. (+1)

6. What describes your reaction to strong bright lights?

    a. I'm not sensitive to bright lights. (+2)

    b. Light has to be very bright for me to notice. (+1)

    c. I'm sensitive to bright lights and prefer sunglasses when outside. (-2)

7. What best describes your tendency toward anxiety or depression?

    a. I tend to become depressed or moody. (+2)

    b. I'm rarely depressed or anxious. (+1)

    c. I tend to become anxious in many situations. (-2)

8. What best describes your current weight?

   a. I am an average weight. (+2)
   b. I am underweight, but can store fat around my waist.
      (-8)
   c. I am overweight or obese. (+6)

9. How do you best describe your appetite?

   a. I live to eat and frequently overeat. (+4)
   b. I use food as fuel, but indulge on occasion. (+2)
   c. I eat to live and sometimes I have to remind myself to
      eat. (-6)

10. What best describes your facial skin?

   a. My skin is very balanced and healthy. (+2)
   b. My skin is sometimes oily and I'm prone to acne or
      breakouts. (+4)
   c. I have sensitive, often dry skin that sometimes looks red
      and irritated. (0)

11. If you needed to stay focused for a long period of time, which
    would help?

   a. Nuts like almonds, walnuts, or peanuts. (+2)
   b. Trail mix with a mix of dried fruit and nuts. (+1)
   c. Dried fruit or candy. (-2)

12. What best describes your digestive system?

   a. I suffer from heartburn or irritable bowel syndrome. (0)
   b. I am frequently constipated or have irregular bowel
      movements. (+4)
   c. I have regular bowel movements with no problems. (+2)

13. What state best describes your energy levels?

    a. I feel mentally balanced, except on rare occasions when I am stressed or don't get enough sleep. (+2)
    b. I feel mentally alert and wired, yet at the same time, physically tired. (-6)
    c. I feel mentally and physically fatigued most of the time. (+4)

14. What happens when you skip meals?

    a. I become irritable, shaky, and/or light-headed. (+4)
    b. I can skip 1 meal and feel fine, but I become irritable, shaky, and/or light-headed if I miss 2 or more meals. (+2)
    c. Skipping meals does not bother me. I frequently go more than 4 to 6 hours without eating. (-4)

15. What best describes your sleeping habits?

    a. I'm frequently tired, but still have difficulty falling asleep and/or getting up in the morning. (+4)
    b. I have difficulty falling asleep or sleeping soundly, yet still feel wired during the day. (-4)
    c. I fall asleep fine, sleep soundly, and wake feeling refreshed. (+2)

16. How do you best describe how old you look?

    a. I look my age. (+1)
    b. I look older than my age. (0)
    c. I look young for my age. (+2)

17. When do you perspire?

   a. I rarely perspire even when exercising. (+2)
   b. I only perspire when exercising or am very hot. (+1)
   c. I perspire a lot during exercise and even when not exercising. (0)

18. How do you best describe your state of awareness and alertness?

   a. I am acutely aware of my surroundings and the people around me, but can find it difficult to focus on any one task. (-4)
   b. It often takes me a moment to register questions and respond. (+2)
   c. I am aware of my surroundings and responsive to people and their questions. (+1)

Total up the number of answers and record them here: _____
Higher than 35: You are a sugar burner.
Between 20 to 35: You are a mixed burner.
Lower than 20: You are a muscle burner.

WHAT KIND OF BURNER ARE YOU?

Sugar Burner

If you scored more than 35, you are a sugar burner.

Sugar burners tend to be overweight, often obese from a young age, and easily develop metabolic resistance. It is very difficult for them to lose fat; the traditional low-calorie diet and aerobic-exercise regimen actually worsens the problem. Sugar burners have a primary defect in insulin metabolism and tend to either overproduce and/or be resistant to the action of this powerful fat-storing hormone.

Sugar burners store fat all over their bodies, not just in one spot. They often look puffy and somewhat waterlogged. Their diets are high in carbohydrates—often up to 70 percent—from pasta, bread, and potatoes. Sugar burners crave sweets, coffee, and chocolate, which may make them feel good for a short 10- to 30-minute spurt, but quickly leave them feeling lethargic and tired. Sugar burners tend to eat constantly. Headaches often occur during exercise. They can have difficulty falling asleep at night and find it just as hard to get out of bed in the morning. Finally, sugar burners tend to be procrastinators, frequently suffer from fatigue and depression, and are at increased risk for diabetes, heart disease, and other illnesses.

○   ○   ○

Judi: A Sugar Burner

At age 35 when Judi looked in the mirror, she no longer saw the lean, muscular athlete she had been in high school and college. She was exhausted all the time, yet couldn't sleep at night. After 4 years of marriage and the birth of two adorable boys, she almost didn't recognize herself. As she looked through pictures from her older son's birthday party, she saw an obese woman she didn't know. Then Judi realized that she *was* that woman. When Judi saw how much weight she had gained and how out of shape she was, she decided to make some serious changes. She cleaned out her refrigerator and cabinets of junk food, dusted off her old stationary bike, and got down to business.

For the next 3 months, Judi watched everything she put in her mouth. She cut back on dietary fat, eating more chicken and fish and less red meat. She measured her whole-grain cereal every morning, added up the calories at every meal, and peppered waitresses with questions whenever she ate out. She exercised for at least an hour a day Monday through Friday, riding her bike, taking long walks through her neighborhood, and even climbing stairs whenever possible to burn more calories.

At the end of 3 months, she stepped on the scale at her doctor's office eager to see the results. When the scale stopped at its final resting place, Judi looked in disbelief. After all that hard work, she had lost only 5 pounds! Barely a dent in the 100 pounds she needed to lose. Judi was in a state of shock. Her sadness quickly turned to anger. She had changed everything. She did not miss a workout, strictly avoided fat, counted all her calories, and had cheated only one time in 3 months by eating half a bagel with cream cheese. Within a few days she was back to her old ways of living and eating away the disappointment of her failure.

When Judi finally came to see us, she was more than 100 pounds overweight at 5 feet, 10 inches, with 45 percent body fat. Although she had nearly given up on finding a way to lose all that weight, she decided to give our short-duration, high-intensity weight training a try.

Judi was clearly a sugar burner. We had her use a fast-paced, 20-minute weight-lifting workout 3 times a week that forced her to rest multiple times during each session. We then gave Judi a pedometer and asked her to walk 15,000 to 20,000 steps a week, about the equivalent of 2 short hikes or daily walking if you live in a city.

Much to Judi's surprise, we told her to eat more, not less, food. Judi was to eat 3 meals, plus 3 snacks a day! It was also important that Judi never allow herself to get hungry. That meant eating fiber-rich snacks, such as fruits and vegetables, to keep the hunger hormone ghrelin down before those hunger pangs set in. Once hunger sets in, the body's internal drive to eat takes over, and the first thing the body wants is something sugary like cookies or some high-fat, high-carb food like pizza. In that case, the body stores fat after a meal. Once Judi started her new regimen, her biggest complaint was that there was too much food and she couldn't finish it! Judi could also have one eat-anything-she-wanted meal once a week—a bowl of pasta, a fast-food burger, 2 scoops of ice cream, or some wine.

After 2 weeks she had lost 10 pounds and slept through the nights. Her Reward Meals became less appealing to her, and with her energy levels back, she started hiking and canoeing with her kids.

The final results? Judi lost more than 100 pounds in a year's time. Best of all, 5 years later, she's kept the weight off, is now strong, trim, and fit, and continues to work the ME program.

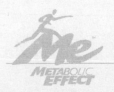

Muscle Burner

If you scored less than 20, you are a muscle burner.

Muscle burners are the envy of their friends. They tend to be thin, even though it seems as if they can eat anything they want. Despite their thin appearance, they have little, if any, muscle tone and loose, sagging skin. We call these people "skinny-fat" because they have a low muscle-to-fat ratio. They burn sugar from muscle tissue due to an oversecretion of the stress hormones cortisol, adrenaline, and noradrenaline. This gives them energy and can often make them high-strung and anxious.

Muscle burners are generally driven, type-A people who are always on the go. They prefer repetitive exercise like running or riding the elliptical trainer, which helps rid them of some nervous energy. They have difficulty staying asleep at night and will sometimes wake repeatedly or sleep very lightly. Muscle burners crave sweets. They may have a few cocktails or wine at the end of the day to calm themselves down. These lifestyle choices can wreak havoc on their bodies. They tend to have weak digestive systems and frequently suffer from irritable bowel syndrome (IBS), ulcers, and gastroesophageal reflux disease. Muscle burners often suffer from anxiety, attention disorders, mood swings, colds and flus, and wild high and low swings in blood sugar.

○ ○ ○

Jessie: A Muscle Burner

Jessie, in her mid-twenties, was thin by anyone's standards. She lived on the treadmill at her local gym and took Pilates classes twice a week. She exercised for at least 1½ hours every day. Her vegetarian diet was simple: cereal and skim milk in the morning. Perhaps hummus, whole-wheat pita, and carrot sticks for lunch. Maybe lentil soup and rice for dinner.

After Jessie's bone density and body fat were measured, her doctor diagnosed her with osteopenia, a condition of weakening bones and a precursor to osteoporosis. Even more puzzling, the amount of her body fat was 29 percent, high for her thin physique. Her doctor referred to her condition as sarcopenic obesity (decreased muscle mass combined with increased subcutaneous fat) and informed Jessie that she didn't have enough muscle. Even Jessie admitted that as thin as she was, her body felt flabby and without tone. Despite her constant running regimen, her arms, butt, and thighs never tightened up.

Concerned that she might have an eating disorder, Jessie was referred to us by her medical doctor. At 5 feet, 7 inches tall and weighing no more than 120 pounds, Jessie's body fat composition was close to 30 percent and she had 87 pounds of lean body mass. She looked anorexic. Think supermodel but a bit heavier. We like to see women with at least 100 pounds of muscle on them, especially if they are taller than 5 feet, 5 inches.

Jessie was upset with how her body looked because she had "no tone, cellulite, and a flat butt." Well, of course she didn't have any muscle tone or an eating disorder; Jessie was running off all her muscle mass! Since she ate no protein, which is essential for muscle mass, she was robbing and burning her muscles to make sugar.

Getting Jessie into the weight room and away from the treadmill took some convincing on our part. She now does 30-minute weight workouts 4 times a week and interval training for 20 minutes on alternate days. No more running as part of her workouts.

Although Jessie is a vegetarian, we call many people like her "carbotarians" because they eat mostly pasta, potatoes, breads, and other carbohydrate-laden foods. By skipping meals, not eating enough protein, and doing all that cardio exercise, Jessie was starving herself by robbing her muscle mass for energy. Her diet now includes eggs, nonfat Greek-style yogurt, whey protein shakes, rice protein shakes, protein bars, and plenty of fruits and vegetables. She occasionally eats chicken and fish. Jessie is allowed 10 to 15 bites of starch with her 3 daily meals. In addition, she can eat 3 to 4 snacks a day.

After 6 months Jessie looked like a different person. She gained 8 pounds and her body fat went down to 22 percent. She added close to 16 pounds of muscle and lost 8 pounds of fat. Lean and toned, Jessie completely transformed her body.

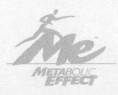

Mixed Burners

If you scored between 20 and 35, then you are a mixed burner.

Mixed burners use sugar and fat as their sources of fuel, and their lifestyle choices largely determine whether they burn sugar or fat. If they stay up too late, they are tired. If they work too hard, they get sick. If they overindulge in food and drink, they gain weight. Most of the people who come to us are mixed burners and their metabolic tendencies are influenced by their chosen lifestyles. High-carbohydrate diets, sedentary lifestyles, and especially stress push these individuals into a sugar-burning state that causes them to gain fat. Menopause and andropause (a loss of male hormones such as testosterone as men age) can also trigger the fat-storing, muscle-burning state. When it comes to food, they can skip meals without feeling hungry, yet often have cravings. The low-calorie diets that worked for them at a younger age lose their effectiveness over time. Calorie-counting diets and aerobic-based exercise programs are effective for a few weeks, but once they stop, the weight they lost returns as quickly as it came off and they regain more fat and lose muscle each time

○ ○ ○

Paul: A Mixed Burner

At 38 years of age, Paul didn't look overweight, but he struggled all his life to keep from gaining weight because obesity and related illnesses such as diabetes ran in his family. He tried to stay in shape by playing golf once a week, running for 30 minutes every so often, or occasionally lifting weights. His chiropractic business was booming—he saw up to fifty patients a day—leaving Paul little time to spend with his wife and kids. He thought he was eating a healthy diet—cereal and juice for breakfast, a sandwich on whole-grain bread or a salad for lunch, and a meat-starch-vegetable dinner, but he often skipped meals, replacing them with lattés, chai tea, bottles of juices, or snacks like chocolate, chips, and pretzels.

Paul said, "If I slack off on my diet at all, I don't feel the same and immediately put on weight. All my diet and exercise efforts are aimed at helping me maintain the status quo. I guess it's all in my genes."

Paul's major issue was a lack of consistency in his exercise program and diet. We see a lot of people like Paul in our line of work, people who think they eat well and exercise regularly, but actually don't. They skip workouts due to other commitments. They make poor food choices because they don't plan their meals ahead or are just too hungry and opt for the wrong kinds of foods.

There was nothing wrong with Paul's genes; he was eating the wrong foods and doing very little fat-burning exercise! He was a typical mixed burner, which means his body used a combination of sugar and fat for its energy. Mixed burners are usually a product of their environments, not their genes. If they eat foods that turn to sugar, their bodies switch their resources to burning sugar instead of fat. When dietary carbohydrate sources are limited and protein intake is increased, they can easily switch to a fat-burning mode.

By changing his workout regimen and food choices, Paul's hormonal signals easily switched into a fat-burning state. Paul did a mixed cardio/ resistance training workout with a certified ME trainer for 15 minutes twice a week. Nothing else. We gave Paul a very simple nutrition plan to follow that focused on quick, satisfying foods such as protein bars, protein shakes, fruit, and nuts he could keep in his office. We encouraged Paul to eat 6 to 7 small meals a day and never let more than a few hours go by between meals and snacks.

By working out twice a week and drastically changing how he ate, Paul lost 29 pounds of fat in 4 months' time.

Now that you've figured out what kind of burner you are—sugar, muscle, or mixed—the next step is to learn what to eat and how to exercise to spark your metabolism and burn fat.

CHAPTER THREE

THE METABOLIC SPARK

Think of your body as a car. When you start it, two things happen: the spark plugs fire and fuel starts to burn. But the spark timing has to be correct and you have to burn the right fuel. You can't burn diesel in a gasoline engine, just as you can't burn gas in a diesel engine.

This concept can be applied to sparking your body's metabolism: you need the right combination of foods (the proper fuel) along with the right exercises (the spark plugs) to trigger your body's fat-burning engine. The two must work together to turn your body into a sustained fat-burning machine. That's the heart of the ME Diet.

The most important thing to realize during the Metabolic Spark Stage is that your metabolism has become used to burning a particular fuel—sugar, muscle, or a combination of the two. Switching into fat-burning mode requires a very deliberate effort aimed at activating the metabolic hormones that drive your body to burn fat.

Your body's ability to burn or not burn fat depends entirely on the choices you make every time you eat and exercise. If you follow the ME program—a high-protein, high-fiber, controlled-carb, low-fat diet and perform the specially designed hybrid exercises—you'll see and feel results in as little as 3 weeks. The better you are about sticking to the ME Diet, the sooner you'll see and feel some very dramatic and positive changes.

By changing your eating habits and exercise routine, the right metabolic messengers are triggered to alter your body's engine. But making just a few adjustments here and there won't work. The only way to shift your body into fat-burning mode is to completely overhaul your diet and exercise choices. The good news is that the changes aren't about deprivation or brutal workouts, and once your new engine is running correctly, you'll find it very easy to maintain.

How do you begin? By integrating new food choices and new exercise habits into your lifestyle. Each time you eat correctly, you'll create a spark in your metabolism. Every exercise session you complete generates a spark. The Metabolic Spark produced by eating specific foods can last several hours and the spark triggered by exercise can last for several days. These sparks create a synergistic effect that triggers your fat-burning engine—and keeps it going. The benefit of these metabolic events is that they keep working and working, even when you're not. The longer you stay with the ME eating and exercise program, the longer the results will last and the more the components will build on one another.

How will you know if your Metabolic Spark has been triggered? You'll suddenly *feel* it. Throughout this phase, your body will be sending you signals about how its metabolism is functioning. For several hours after each meal, you will feel energetic, satisfied, and focused, with no hunger pangs or discomfort. Cravings for sweets and stimulants will dissipate. The exercise sessions will release yet another set of metabolic messengers that will further trigger your metabolic processes, heighten your sense of awareness, and elevate your mood. You'll feel a satisfying soreness in your muscles as well as some tightening of the connective tissues surrounding your joints. Within a few short weeks, you'll experience an elevated sense of vibrancy and begin to see physical changes in your body. You may notice a slight amount of weight loss along with an increased firmness and tone of some muscles. Muscle contour may begin to show as well. The ultimate effect is different for everyone and depends on your own metabolic makeup and how committed you are to the necessary food and exercise choices.

FOOD: A NEW APPROACH

The ME nutritional program is tailored to your unique, individual metabolic needs to support your best hormonal balance. Listen to your hunger, cravings, and energy levels to tell you how to sense and evaluate the hormonal balance created by the foods you eat. A perfect metabolic meal will leave you satisfied and with focused energy for longer periods of time. You know those nagging cravings for salt, sugar, chocolate, and caffeine? They'll be fewer and much more manageable. You'll also be more tuned in to your metabolic sensations. We have found that the following tips help people achieve their Metabolic Effect:

Do not skip meals or snacks. Skipping meals causes the body to secrete stress hormones like adrenaline and cortisol, and then insulin. This combination of hormones puts the body into a muscle-burning rather than a fat-burning mode. Skipping meals also causes an imbalance in brain chemistry that leads to binge eating later in the day. When hunger sets in, your brain sends signals that say, "Feed me. Now!" You're unwilling to wait until dinner is cooked or until all those salad vegetables are washed, dried, and ready to toss. So, you stuff your mouth with some crackers or cookies or a candy bar—anything to take away that gnawing hunger—undoing all the hard work you've done. Breakfast is indeed the most important meal of the day because it establishes the proper hormonal fat-burning rhythms for the day. Pay attention to how you feel when you eat breakfast as well as to what you eat. Breakfast should be consumed within the first two hours after waking up.

Eat every 2 to 4 hours. Never let more than four hours go by without eating and never let yourself get hungry. This is why we suggest specific snacks in our program. Once you become hungry, your body will instinctively seek out sweet, starchy, processed foods for immediate gratification. This concept may seem like heresy to a calorie counter, but from the fat-burning perspective, you need to eat so you are constantly and consistently sending the right signals to burn fat.

Do not eat for at least 2 hours before going to sleep for the night. Perhaps the biggest weakness in the calorie-counting approach to weight loss happens at night. If you deprive yourself of food all day long, the body will set countermeasures in motion that relentlessly drive you to find food. This is why countless dieters usually break down at night and cannot go to sleep without something sweet. To achieve the Metabolic Spark, do just the opposite. Go to bed on an empty stomach, avoiding all food for at least 2 hours before turning in. For most people, the last meal or snack of the day should be consumed no later than eight P.M. Sleep can be a prime fat-burning time or a prime fat-storing time. Your choices about what to eat and how late to eat directly affect this. If you eat late at night, then the chances are that you will be storing fat as you sleep rather than burning it.

Prepare ahead of time when it comes to food, especially snacks. Put ½-cup servings of nuts in small plastic bags and keep them with you—in your handbag, in your desk drawer, in your car. Wash and cut up salad greens and vegetables and make fruit salad as soon as you bring your purchases home from the market so they're ready to eat when hunger knocks. Keep your blender clean and ready to use, and have ingredients nearby for quick protein smoothies.

COFFEE AND OTHER STIMULANTS

No, you don't have to give up your morning cup of joe, but know that coffee comes with some risks as well as some surprising benefits. Coffee is loaded with phytochemicals and is the major dietary source of perhaps the best-known plant chemical of all, caffeine. Caffeine raises the stress hormones cortisol, adrenaline, and noradrenaline.

What's interesting is how caffeine affects sugar burners. One cup of strong caffeinated coffee before exercising can actually *increase* the fat-burning effects of a sugar burner's workout. If you drink a cup of coffee and don't exercise, the caffeine will increase stress hormone production and lead to metabolic resistance. While just a small amount of coffee triggers this reaction in sugar burners, coffee has this effect on all burner types in varying degrees. Don't think you can fool your body into burning more fat by drinking more coffee—it won't work. Instead, your body will develop tolerance and adrenal hormone resistance. Coffee is not something that should be used indiscriminately for a fat-burning diet. The bottom line: sugar and mixed burners may benefit from one cup of coffee before a workout, but muscle burners are better off not drinking coffee.

Yes, it's hard to give up, but know that coffee creates a stress-hormone release that can send some people into an unbalanced metabolic state, leading to increased hunger throughout the day and even more cravings at night. Many people are unaware that their nighttime cravings and insatiable desire to eat are directly related to the coffee they drank in the morning. If this sounds familiar, then reduce your consumption of coffee as much as possible; drink green or black tea, or try cocoa instead. If you can't live without coffee, learn to drink it black accompanied by high-protein/high-fiber foods or just before a workout. This allows the stress response to be countered by the fat-burning and growth-promoting effects of certain foods and exercise.

By the way, decaffeinated coffee often has the same effect as regular coffee. For some people, just the taste of coffee can be enough to create a hormonal stress response.

Stimulants like coffee, tea, and sodas affect hormonal function and fat burning. When used in conjunction with intense exercise, coffee can often be a benefit for certain metabolic types. But for others, it can lead to a further imbalance in hormonal metabolism. The problem with coffee and other caffeinated substances is that they release stress hormones and stored sugar (glycogen) into the bloodstream and create a fight-or-flight reaction that floods the body with blood sugar. If the blood sugar isn't used, the body then responds by secreting insulin to rebalance the blood sugar. This, as you have learned, is the antithesis of fat burning.

High cortisol levels along with high insulin levels bring fat burning to a standstill and increase cravings for sweet and fatty foods. Muscle burners who already have an excess stress hormone secretion will be thrown even further out of balance by drinking coffee. Mixed burners seem to do fine with stimulants—1 cup of black coffee or tea in the morning— as long as they aren't consumed too often. Sugar burners can also use stimulants to their advantage if consumed in moderation.

COUNT BITES OF CARBS/STARCHES

Having worked with thousands of people, we realize that everyone just wants to sit down and enjoy a meal without carrying a calculator or a measuring cup, or worrying about being on a diet. Who has time to measure and weigh food, or total up the number of calories consumed? That's why we came up with a simple way to measure limited foods such as carbohydrate-rich starches: count bites.

We use the bite-counting concept because most people have a fairly consistent amount of food they consume with each bite. Think of a bite as the typical amount of food you would place in your mouth if you were eating with a spoon. If you are someone who absolutely requires an amount, then a bite according to our rule is 1 level tablespoon.

Use this rule for certain foods depending on what type of burner you are, but in general this rule applies to carbohydrate-rich starches. Once you know the number of bites you should have with each meal, it will take you about 1 to 2 weeks before you instinctively know exactly how much of a starch to eat.

Counting bites has several advantages. It slows you down so that you are more conscious of your meal and are less likely to eat too much. Counting bites gets you out of the calorie-counting mind-set and, instead, lets you focus on the amounts and ratios of foods you are eating. The most beneficial aspect of counting bites is that it is easy to remember and easy to practice. You can go anywhere and know exactly how much to eat without pulling out a calorie-counting booklet.

DO I HAVE TO EAT THE STARCH BITES?

Many of our clients ask if they can skip eating the bites of starchy food altogether. We don't recommend this for most people. Avoiding carbohydrates entirely may lead to increased hunger and cravings along with lower energy levels. Use the bite rule to fine-tune your diet for your specific metabolism.

If your hunger, craving, and energy levels are stable, then decreasing the amount of carbohydrate bites can be a good strategy for quicker results. If, however, your energy levels falter and/or your cravings and hunger levels rise, even after you have increased the amount of fiber and protein at each meal, start by eating 2 more starch bites per meal until cravings and hunger levels are stabilized. By paying close attention to how you feel, you can decide whether to increase or decrease your number of starch bites at each meal to maintain your energy and speed up fat loss. Remember that sweet fruits and alcohol count as starch bites. Following the suggestions on your metabolic plate will he help you zero in on the Metabolic Diet perfectly suited to you.

Starchy Carbohydrate Choices

If you are a *sugar* burner, you may have *3 to 5* bites of one of the following starches.

If you are a *mixed* burner, you may have *5 to 10* bites of one of the following starches.

If you are a *muscle* burner, you may have *7 to 15* bites of one of the following starches.

Vegetables: artichokes, leeks, lima beans, okra, squash (acorn, butternut, pumpkin), sweet potatoes or yams, and turnips

Legumes: black beans, adzuki beans, chickpeas, cowpeas, Great Northern beans, kidney beans, lentils, mung beans, navy beans, pinto beans, split peas, white beans

Grains: barley, brown rice, buckwheat groats (kasha), bulgur (tabbouleh), millet, polenta, steel-cut oats, and tapioca

Breads and crackers: whole-grain breads, whole-grain cooked cereals, ak-mak crackers, Ezekiel bread, Wasa crackers, and whole-grain tortillas

Notice that this list includes only certain vegetables, whole grains, legumes, and beans. There are no "white" starches such as white rice, cookies, saltines, sweets, and other processed foods. The reason is that these foods should be limited as much as possible. That is why your bites are listed in a range. The whiter the starch, the fewer bites you should take and the smaller they should be. For example, if you are a mixed burner and choose to eat white bread with dinner, then limit yourself to 5 small bites at each meal. However, if you opt for brown rice instead, you can enjoy 10 bigger bites. In this way, you can easily regulate the hormonal influence of your meals.

VEGETABLES

When it comes to the following vegetables, eat as many of them as you wish no matter what type of burner you are. Salad greens, tomatoes, herbs, and some other vegetables can be enjoyed raw, but others are best when steamed or roasted. Keep vegetables cut up and ready for snacking and cooking.

- arugula
- asparagus
- bamboo shoots
- bean sprouts
- beet greens
- bell peppers (red, yellow, green)
- broad beans
- broccoli
- brussels sprouts
- cabbage
- cassava
- cauliflower
- celery
- chayote fruit
- chicory
- chives
- collard greens
- coriander
- cucumber
- dandelion greens
- eggplant
- endive
- fennel
- garlic
- gingerroot
- green beans
- hearts of palm
- jicama (raw)
- jalapeño peppers
- kale
- kohlrabi
- lettuce
- mushrooms
- mustard greens
- onions
- parsley
- radicchio
- radishes
- snap beans
- snow peas
- shallots
- spinach
- spaghetti squash
- summer squash
- swiss chard
- tomatoes
- turnip greens
- watercress

FRUIT

Whether you're a sugar, muscle, or mixed burner, you can eat unlimited quantities of certain fruits. Enjoy fresh fruit whenever possible. You can use frozen fruit for smoothies, but never canned fruits, which are usually packed in sugar-loaded syrups.

If you are a sugar burner, you can eat unlimited quantities of:

- apples
- berries (blackberries, blueberries, boysenberries, gooseberries, loganberries, raspberries, strawberries)
- cherries
- grapefruit
- lemons
- limes
- pears

If you are a mixed burner, you can eat unlimited amounts of the above fruits as well as:

- apricots
- avocados
- kiwifruit
- all melons except watermelon
- nectarines
- oranges
- passion fruit
- peaches
- persimmons
- plums
- pomegranates
- prunes
- tangerines

If you're a muscle burner, you can eat unlimited amounts of the above fruits as well as:

- bananas
- grapes
- mango
- papaya
- pineapple
- watermelon

If you eat fruits that are not on your list, that's fine, but then you must treat them as if they're starches and limit them to your specific bite rule to keep you in an elevated fat-burning state. For example, if you're a sugar burner who loves bananas, have just 3 to 5 small bites per meal and forgo any additional starch. Eventually, knowing which fruits are good for you and which should be limited will become second nature.

○ ○ ○

Smoothies

For breakfast or an in-between-meals snack, nothing beats a fruity, delicious protein-packed smoothie. Protein-based smoothies are a great way to keep hunger at bay, build muscle, and burn fat.

We prefer whey protein powder, a dairy by-product, which is available in any health food store. Good-tasting (they are available in many flavors) whey protein powder is inexpensive and lowers cortisol (see page 116). It is excellent for building muscle mass and is a complete source of protein. (Metabolic Effect, Jay Robb, and Designer Whey are three brands we recommend.) If you're a vegetarian, look for a rice-based protein powder. Use soy-based protein powders sparingly since some of them have been shown to have negative hormonal effects, specifically regarding thyroid and testosterone activity. Whey protein powders are available everywhere—health food, vitamin, and warehouse stores; supermarkets; and drugstores.

For one serving, put 1 to 2 scoops (each container comes with its own scoop) whey protein powder and one cup (8 ounces) liquid, choosing from water, skim milk, unsweetened almond milk, or coconut water (not coconut milk) in the blender. Coconut water is packed with replenishing electrolytes. (Again, we avoid soy milk for the reasons above.) Add the specific fruits and flavorings as indicated below along with 1 teaspoon fiber powder such as acacia fiber powder or apple pectin powder (available online or in health food stores) or ME Fiber Complex™. These are soluble fibers derived from fruits and vegetables that help slow food transit through the body, decrease fat absorption, blunt a fast rise in glucose, and lower the hunger hormones CCK and ghrelin. Add a handful of ice cubes to the blender. Blend and drink immediately.

You can add an optional scoop of ME Recovery Greens™ or ME Recovery Reds™ to smoothies for additional nutrition, especially if you don't eat enough vegetables and fruits in their natural form. Avoid greens powders that contain grasses and fillers. ME Recovery Greens™ are made with pure organic vegetables like broccoli, cauliflower, chard, kale, cauliflower, and others and have a lemon-lime flavor with a touch of sweetness from stevia. ME Recovery Reds™ contain powdered blueberries, cherries, pomegranates, and apples.

If you like your smoothie with a bit of sweetness, there are several natural sweeteners that can be used in place of refined sugar, honey, or artificial sweeteners. Zero-carb, zero-calorie stevia, also known as sweet leaf, is made from an herb originally grown in South America. Stevia is available in tablet, liquid, or powder form. A little bit goes a long way; stevia extracts can be up to three hundred times sweeter than the same amount of sugar. Just a drop or two in your smoothie will add plenty of sweetness. Stevia is readily available in supermarkets and health food stores. Truvia is just one brand name for stevia. Other types of healthy sweeteners include xylitol (XyloSweet) and erythritol (Zero and Sweet Simplicity).

Here are ten easy ideas, but feel free to create your own smoothies. There are more smoothie recipes starting on page 181.

Berry Good Smoothie: Use skim milk or unsweetened almond milk. Add ¼ banana and ½ to 1 cup frozen or fresh blueberries, strawberries, or raspberries.

Banana-Chocolate Smoothie: Use skim milk or unsweetened almond milk. Add ¼ banana and 1 teaspoon cocoa powder.

Banana-Coconut Smoothie: Use 4 ounces coconut water and 4 ounces light coconut milk. Add ¼ banana.

Chocolate–Peanut Butter Smoothie: Use skim milk or unsweetened almond milk. Add ¼ banana, 1 tablespoon creamy peanut butter, and 1 teaspoon cocoa powder.

Coconut-Pineapple Smoothie: Use light coconut milk. Add ½ cup frozen pineapple chunks.

Green Monster: Use water and strawberry-flavored whey protein. Add 2 tablespoons ME Recovery Greens™, ¼ banana, and ½ cup strawberries.

Pecan Pie Smoothie: Use coconut water. Add ¼ banana and 1 handful shelled pecans.

Spice Smoothie: Use coconut water. Add 1 handful shelled walnuts, a pinch of cinnamon, a pinch of nutmeg, and ½ teaspoon maple extract.

Tropical Fruit Smoothie: Use skim milk or unsweetened almond milk. Add ½ cup frozen mango or pineapple chunks.

Vanilla Smoothie: Use skim milk and unsweetened almond milk. Add ½ teaspoon vanilla extract.

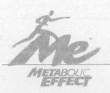

PROTEIN

Eating protein has major implications for hormonal balance. Protein helps control cravings and hunger; aids in generating glucagon, a hormone/metabolic messenger that increases the use of fat for energy; and is required for maintaining muscle mass by providing amino acid building blocks. Protein is the second most abundant substance in the body besides water, and the more you are able to use it to build muscle, the leaner, tighter, and firmer you will become.

Many people incorrectly think of protein in terms of total amount needed to keep from becoming protein deficient. But metabolism works in ratios. The fat-burning outcome of a meal is largely determined by the ratio of protein to carbohydrate, because proteins initiate the release of the fat-burning hormone glucagon, while carbohydrates cause the secretion of fat-storing insulin. When choosing protein sources, it is essential that you pay close attention to this ratio.

Many foods, including beans, legumes, nuts, seeds, and dairy products, are perceived as being great protein sources, but fall short when the hormonal effects are analyzed. While beans do have more protein than most other plant foods, their carbohydrate content is more than 70 percent starch! This means that when beans are ingested, the insulin signal is magnified to a greater degree than glucagon's signal. Nuts and seeds also have protein, but are high in fat and lack the necessary potent fat-burning punch. Many milk products are also a less than desirable protein for fat burning but are superior to nuts and beans. The amino acids that make up milk and cheese are potent stimulators of insulin. This is in spite of the low glycemic index of dairy. Muscle burners can eat dairy products such as milk and cheese, and mixed burners can handle small amounts, but sugar burners should eat milk products sparingly if at all.

The best protein sources are foods that contain mostly protein and have little starch or fat. These include all types of lean animal protein, especially chicken, turkey, pork, and beef, as well as eggs, game meats (venison, buffalo, elk, etc.), and fish. Wild-caught fish, farm raised game meat, and organic animal protein are best.

Soy is a popular protein choice among nonmeat eaters, but is not the best choice for fat burning. Soy acts as a weak estrogen and therefore can interfere with the fat-burning effects of testosterone, which is important for men and women. In addition, soy negatively impacts enzymes required to make the thyroid hormone, which is a major fat-burning hormone. Soy is also a common allergen.

Protein is often given a bad rap in the same way that both fat and carbohydrates were singled out as "bad foods." Protein has been shown to enhance muscle mass and bone density as well as speed fat burning. It has also been shown to improve cholesterol profiles and, contrary to popular myth, increased protein in the diet does not cause problems with the kidneys or liver and actually helps keep them healthier.

VEGETARIANS, VEGANS, AND THE ME DIET

Vegetarians and vegans do very well with the ME Diet. As a matter of fact, vegetarians and vegans have a leg up on meat eaters in some ways because they have already learned one of the cardinal rules of metabolic eating—eat lots of fruits and vegetables.

The challenge is to increase the protein content and reduce the amount of grains in the typical vegetarian diet. Vegetarian sources of protein often contain a much higher proportion of sugar than protein. It's the protein-to-starch ratio that determines a food's hormonal effect. Ovo-lacto vegetarians do well on the ME program when they increase their intake of eggs and dairy (milk, cheese, yogurt) and can use whey protein. When these higher-protein foods replace grains and beans and the usually high fruit and vegetable intake is increased even more, the high-fiber, high-phytonutrient, protein-rich Metabolic Effect Diet is easily followed.

For vegans, it's absolutely essential to include vegan protein powders in your diet and avoid the "carbotarian" mentality of eating more grains than fruits and vegetables. We recommend rice, hemp, and nut protein powders over soy, but for vegans soy is a much better option than eliminating protein altogether or relying on starches like beans for protein.

REWARD MEALS

When most people think of eating healthy, the word "diet" comes to mind. But as we've explained, diets usually don't work because they tend to go against our body's inherent feast-or-famine response. As you decrease your food intake when dieting, the body responds with a lowering of metabolism and a slow drop in the hunger hormone leptin. This is good for a short period of time, perhaps 3 to 5 days, but if calorie deprivation continues for a week, it will eventually cause raging hunger and relentless food cravings. (That's why the first few days of a calorie-counting diet seem so easy!)

This hormonal-driven event is an ancient human survival mechanism that remains with us today. It was the ideal survival tool for early humans who had no guarantees as to where their next meal would come from and how substantial it would be.

Research shows that one high-calorie meal per week has the ability to reset the hormonal hunger signals sent by leptin and ghrelin (another hunger hormone). By allowing yourself to eat one meal with as much and whatever foods you like, you can exert control over your body's hunger thermostat. Depending on your metabolic type and your progress with the ME Diet, you will be able to enjoy between 1 to 3 Reward Meals per week.

Reward Meals are an important component of a fat-loss diet. Your body is designed to efficiently seek out high-calorie foods, including fat and sugar, whenever you begin to regulate food intake in any way. Sticking to a high-fiber, higher-protein diet works to dramatically blunt this effect, but eating other foods, specifically carbohydrates, one meal a week works to circumvent the body's natural food-regulating behaviors.

As you eat and the body begins to burn fat, your hunger hormones will normalize, reversing the metabolic resistance that has occurred over the years of eating for weight loss instead of fat loss. At some point they will signal the body to begin eating once again, causing increased hunger and cravings. Usually, eating frequent small meals, focusing on large amounts of fiber and increasing protein, stops this effect. It's actually beneficial to raise the hunger hormones by eating a high-carb, high-calorie meal once a week after several days of adhering to a fat-loss plan.

Usually one high-carb, high-calorie meal is all it will take to dramatically reset those hunger hormones. Depending on your type and progression through the metabolic effect, you'll learn to use these Reward Meals strategically. You'll have one Reward Meal each week in the Spark Stage no matter what kind of burner you are. Mixed burners should keep their Reward Meals at 1 per week during the Spark and Transformation Stages, progressing to 2 Reward Meals per week during the Metabolic Effect Stage. Sugar burners should limit their Reward Meals to 1 meal per week no matter what phase they are in. Muscle burners can add one Reward Meal per week at each stage of the program. These meals can be eaten all in one day, but are better if consumed several days apart, such as on Wednesday and Saturday nights. They are also most advantageous when consumed within 2 hours of an ME Workout.

Indulging once a week in favorite foods also serves a psychological purpose. Food is something to savor and enjoy, and while some people eat to live, others live to eat. Consistently denying yourself the occasional treat or a great restaurant meal will only make you resentful, so we urge our clients to eat whatever they want at 1 meal a week. A steak dinner with all the sides and some good red wine. Pancakes or waffles with bacon for breakfast. A cheeseburger and fries for lunch. Another benefit of eating as much food as you like once a week is how you will feel after your weekly indulgence. That once-familiar lethargic, heavy feeling will return along with possible digestive disturbances, headaches, and other nagging physical symptoms that most people live with but never connect with the food they eat. Clients are always eager to get back on track.

You will gladly return to your fat-burning diet after that all-you-can-eat meal, because you'll quickly feel the difference. You'll miss those increased energy levels—not the wired feeling of being on coffee—but the steady, sustained energy that only a balanced metabolism can bring. Frequent hunger pangs and cravings will dissipate. A mental focus and clarity also comes with this way of eating, along with a noticeable improvement in your sleep pattern. These effects usually precede the rapid change in body composition that follows.

Your once-a-week treat should provide both enjoyment as well as a reminder of how powerful the hormonal influences of food are.

○ ○ ○

Listening to Your Body

As holistic physicians, we look at symptoms differently from most doctors. To us, symptoms are clues to how your body is functioning in the world. You're as different from everyone else biochemically as you are physically. To tune in to those differences, listen to the powerful clues your body sends you, such as fatigue when you're hungry, cravings, sleep disturbances, recovery from workouts, and other factors. They're expressions of your metabolic process and hormonal balance that can aid you when it comes to metabolic balance and fat burning.

If you're eating well, sleeping through the night, doing your workouts, and paying attention to all the other lifestyle tips we mention, then your body is burning its fat stores effectively. If you're hungry and have cravings, then you need to eat regularly and frequently and use the guidelines on your individual plate to adjust protein and fiber intake. If you're still hungry and craving food, slowly increase the number of starch bites to balance out your metabolic processes. Listen to your body and make the appropriate adjustments based on your unique metabolic makeup. It's a powerful feeling.

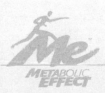

THE ME PLATES: WHAT TO EAT

Based on your answers to the questionnaire, we can get a good idea of what type of fuel your body prefers to burn for energy—sugar, fat, or both. Sugar is derived from several sources—the food you eat, stored sugar called glycogen, or the amino acids from muscle tissue that can burn as sugar. Although the body burns both sugar and fat all the time, the relative ratios of each make a huge difference in body composition.

People have a natural tendency toward burning a particular fuel, determined to some degree by genetics, but what fuel is burned is also tremendously impacted by early childhood eating patterns and every-day food choices. Most people burn sugar preferentially over fat because the food they eat, the type of exercise they do, and the lifestyle they live forces their metabolic machinery to run primarily on sugar and preferentially store fat. But not all sugar burners are equal. Some are able to use sugar they have stored and will be less likely to break down muscle to make sugar. Others will break down muscle tissue as a primary means of supplying the body with sugar. And still others will be able to burn sugar along with a mix of muscle and fat.

By knowing what your fuel-burning tendencies are, it is easy to manipulate food choices to trigger those fat-burning hormones.

What to Eat If You're a Sugar Burner

If you are a sugar burner, your body has become very inefficient at burning fat for energy and relies almost exclusively on sugar. This is because the predominant hormone balance in a sugar burner turns off fat-burning enzymes while enhancing sugar-burning and fat-storing enzymes. Your hormonal situation is likely one in which cortisol and insulin are elevated to the point of hormone resistance, making you a very inefficient user of fat and forcing your body to burn sugar instead. Along with this, your body is probably not getting the signal the hunger hormone leptin is sending. You feel hungry all the time and have frequent cravings for foods rich in sugar and fat. Diabetes and other hormonal disorders, including hypothyroidism, may run in your family.

The good news is that you probably have plenty of muscle on your frame. Good because muscle tissue is a prime mover of hormonal metabolism. Once you begin to exercise and eat appropriately, you will trigger your hormonal fat-burning machinery. To turn your body's fat-burning machinery on, you have to switch your hormones back into a fat-burning balance. The best way to do this is to slowly force the body to use its fat, an impossible task if you keep feeding the body sugar. The body burns what you feed it. Switch your nutritional choices to protein, fiber, and the right fats and the body will shift from using sugar to burning fat. This, along with tailored hormonal exercise, will change your metabolism for good.

Every single time you eat according to this plate, you will set into motion a hormonal software program that will elevate fat burning in the body. Eat plenty of food—meals and snacks—and don't allow yourself to get ravenously hungry. Focus on lean protein, lots of vegetables, low-sugar fruits, and very little starch and sugar.

- Eat 3 meals and 3 snacks every day. Eat small meals every 2 to 3 hours.
- Eat as many vegetables as you like, with no limit. Eat as much of the following fruit as you like: All berries (blueberries, raspberries, blackberries, strawberries, cherries), apples, and pears according to your food list. Avoid sweet fruits such as pineapples, oranges, bananas, mangoes, grapes, and watermelon. Eat more vegetables than fruit.
- Eat as much lean animal protein as you like—chicken, egg whites, fish, turkey, beef, Canadian bacon. Buy wild, cold-water fish—not farm-raised—such as salmon, halibut, cod, mackerel, and tuna, and organic poultry and beef whenever possible.

- Eat no more than 3 to 5 bites of starchy carbohydrates per meal. The whiter the starch, the fewer bites you should have and the smaller they should be.
- Eat no more than ½ cup of nuts or 1 to 2 tablespoons of nut butter per day. Choose from almonds, walnuts, unsalted peanuts, and Brazil nuts.
- Snack on beef or venison jerky, protein bars, protein shakes, and vegetables.
- Consume limited quantities of cheese—2 tablespoons of crumbled feta cheese on a salad or 2 tablespoons of grated Parmesan on grilled chicken—milk, yogurt, and other dairy products. Think of these as condiments.
- Enjoy a Reward Meal once a week, choosing whatever and as much food as you want.
- Avoid alcohol, beer, and wine except at your once-a-week Reward meal. If you choose to drink alcohol, then skip the starch and limit consumption to 3 to 5 sips.
- Between meals and snacks pay attention to hunger, cravings, and energy levels. Adjust meals and snacks accordingly to balance these hormonal indicators.

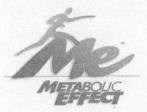

The
Sugar-Burner's
Plate

Eat 4–6 Meals Daily

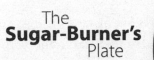

2–3 Different Vegetables
& /or Fruit

Lean Protein
(keeping dairy to a minimum)

Starchy Carbs & Sweet Fruits
3–5 Bites

* Between each meal track the following:

1. Hunger .... ▼ ▲ Ø
2. Energy .... ▼ ▲ Ø
3. Cravings .... ▼ ▲ Ø

▲ = High or Increased

Ø = No Change or Normal

▼ = Low or Decreased

What to Eat If You're a Mixed Burner

As a mixed sugar and fat burner, you have an advantage over sugar burners and muscle burners. By changing what you eat, your hormonal signals can trigger a fat-burning mode. You naturally have a well-regulated metabolism, are probably neither too thin nor overweight, and have a good amount of muscle on your body.

Mixed burners are usually products of their environment and can quickly adapt to other lifestyles. You have a steady amount of energy, so focus on getting a good balance of nutrients from lean protein sources, healthy fats, and a wide array of fruits and vegetables.

To push your metabolism into a higher state of fat burning, you will need to regulate your metabolic fire with sugar/starch foods that are burned slowly while providing plenty of protein to maintain your muscle mass. Enjoy old-fashioned oatmeal, brown rice, and baked potatoes with their skins. Avoid bread, pasta, and sweets.

Every time you eat according to this plate, you set into motion a hormonal software program that will raise the fat-burning mechanism in your body.

- Eat as many vegetables as you like, with no limit. Eat as many fruits as you like except the very sweet fruits (banana, pineapple, watermelon, mango, grapes). See your food list.
- Eat as much lean animal protein as you like—chicken, egg whites, fish, turkey, beef, Canadian bacon. Buy wild fish—not farm-raised—and organic poultry and beef whenever possible.
- Eat starch and sugar according to bites. Eat no more than 5 to 10 bites of starchy carbohydrates per meal. The whiter the starch, the fewer bites you should have and the smaller they should be.
- Eat up to 1 cup of nuts or 2 tablespoons of nut butter per day. Choose from almonds, walnuts, peanuts, and Brazil nuts.

- Eat 3 meals and 2 to 4 snacks every day.
- Snack on beef or venison jerky, protein bars, protein shakes, and vegetables.
- Enjoy a Reward Meal once a week, choosing whatever and as much as you want.
- Use dairy products as a condiment—2 tablespoons yogurt with fruit salad, nonfat milk in your coffee, etc.
- Avoid alcohol, beer, and wine except at your once-a-week Reward Meal. If you choose to have alcohol, then skip the starch and limit consumption to 5 to 10 sips.
- Between meals and snacks pay attention to hunger, cravings, and energy levels. Adjust meals and snacks accordingly to balance these hormonal indicators.

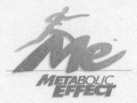

The
Mixed-Burner's
Plate

Eat 4–6 Meals Daily

2–3 Different
Vegetables
& /or Fruit

Lean Protein
(keeping dairy to
a minimum)

Starchy Carbs
& Sweet Fruits

5–10 Bites

* Between each meal track the following:

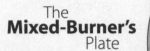

1. Hunger _ _ _ _ _ _ _ _ _ _ ▼ ▲ Ø
2. Energy _ _ _ _ _ _ _ _ _ _ ▼ ▲ Ø
3. Cravings _ _ _ _ _ _ _ _ _ ▼ ▲ Ø

▲ = High or Increased

Ø = No Change or Normal

▼ = Low or Decreased

What to Eat If You're a Muscle Burner

Although your body type burns sugar for energy, muscles, rather than food, supply the fuel. Muscle burners are often high-strung type-A people who seem to run on "nervous energy." They release a larger amount of the stress hormones cortisol and adrenaline. Muscle burners tend to be thin in their youth, but often develop what is called the "skinny-fat" look, in which they appear to be thin though their bodies are flabby, with an unfavorable muscle-to-fat ratio. Any pronounced fat storage is concentrated around the belly. This look is often seen in models, actors, and long-distance runners. They often skip breakfast.

Muscle burners can often go for long periods—from 3 to 6 hours—without eating, may suffer from anxiety, and may have been considered underweight much of their lives. Diabetes, loose connective tissue, and degenerative disorders such as osteoporosis, arthritis, sarcopenia (loss of muscle mass), and fibromyalgia are often consequences for muscle burners who yo-yo diet and don't eat properly.

Muscle burners need to balance out the biochemical overdrive created by the adrenal hormones adrenaline, noradrenaline, and cortisol. High amounts of these hormones break down muscle tissue to supply the body with sugar. While it's important to consume enough sugar to slow the adrenal hormone burst and feed the body, it's just as crucial to eat a balanced diet of protein and fat for a steady supply of energy. That is why eating breakfast is so important. Once the nutritional hormonal inputs are corrected, the body will begin to spare its muscle stores and burn fat more readily, leading to an overall toned body and more consistent energy.

Every single time you eat according to this plate, you will set into motion a hormonal software program that will elevate fat burning in the body. Eat as many vegetables and fruits as you like with no limit.

- Eat as much lean animal protein as you like—chicken, egg whites, fish, turkey, beef, Canadian bacon. Buy wild fish—

not farm-raised—and organic poultry and beef whenever possible.

- Eat no more than 7 to 15 bites of starchy carbohydrates at each meal. If you're eating sweet white starches, limit consumption to 7 bites.
- Eat up to 1½ cups of nuts or 3 tablespoons of nut butter per day.
- Eat 3 meals and at least 3 snacks every day.
- Snack on beef or venison jerky, protein bars, protein shakes, and vegetables.
- Enjoy a Reward Meal (see page 56) once a week, choosing whatever and as much as you want.
- Enjoy low-fat dairy products such as cheese, yogurt, and skim milk.
- Avoid alcohol, beer, and wine except at your once-a-week Reward Meal. If you choose to have alcohol, then skip the starch altogether and limit consumption to 7 to 15 sips.
- Between meals and snacks pay attention to hunger, cravings, and energy levels. Adjust meals and snacks accordingly to balance these hormonal indicators.

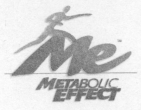

The
Muscle-Burner's
Plate

Eat 4–6 Meals Daily

2–3 Different Vegetables & /or Fruit

Lean Protein
(keeping dairy to a minimum)

Starchy Carbs
7–15 Bites

* Between each meal track the following:

1. Hunger ▼ ▲ Ø
2. Energy ▼ ▲ Ø
3. Cravings ▼ ▲ Ø

▲ = High or Increased

Ø = No Change or Normal

▼ = Low or Decreased

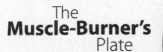

ADJUST USING THIS GUIDE

If Hunger ▲ = ▲ Fiber & ▲ Protein, ▲ H20
If Cravings ▲ = ▲ Fiber & ▲ Protein, ▲ Exercise, ▲ Sleep

If ▼ Energy = ▲ Fiber, ▲ Protein

CHAPTER FOUR
THE METABOLIC SPARK WORKOUT

THE HYBRID EXERCISES

Many people wrongly assume that exercise is about how long you work out. They think the longer you work out, the more calories you burn. Or they are concerned—particularly women—that if they lift weights, they will "bulk up" and look like bodybuilders.

To see real results, you need to work harder and increase the amount of energy expended during your workout. A shorter, harder workout also means you will spend far less time in the gym. The ME Workout does this by condensing both interval training and weight training into 1 compact full-body, 30-minute workout.

What are the differences between interval and weight training? Interval training is a form of cardiovascular training that alternates intense bursts of activity with less strenuous active rest periods. An example would be a 30-second sprint on a bike followed by 1 minute of slow motion pedaling to recover and catch your breath before repeating the intense 30-second sprint. Athletes have trained like this for years! Think about it, 90 percent of all sports—tennis, basketball, hockey, volleyball—alternate periods of intense activity with periods of lower intensity. Weight or resistance training is strength training with each exercise performed against an opposing force by using resistance. This resistance can come from free weights like dumbbells or bars, machines such as those made by Cybex, rubber resistance bands, or even your own body weight. The ME Workout uses dumbbells because they are versatile and provide a unique challenge to all of your muscles, including the stabilizing muscles in your core, legs, and upper body.

A study in the *Journal of Strength and Conditioning Research* (September 2008) showed that a workout that alternates cardiovascular bursts and heavy weight training burned nine times more fat than the same workout done by separating the cardio from the weights. This study also showed that muscle gains, strength, endurance, and aerobic capacity improved when the two workouts were mixed together. In an earlier study (January 2008 in the same journal), the same condensed workout reduced the time it took to recover from postexercise muscle soreness. Why does the ME Workout improve results, save time, and speed recovery? Not because more calories are burned, but because the ME Workout produces an accelerated metabolic afterburn that leads to increased energy usage for 16 to 48 hours after the workout, ensuring that the energy burned is from fat, not sugar.

The first stage of the ME Workout helps you get used to the unique hybrid-style exercises and kicks your metabolism into fat-burning gear. To find your appropriate weights, choose a dumbbell that allows you to do 3 perfect bicep curls, not 2, not 4, but 3. Then divide the number of pounds in that weight by half. That is the amount of weight you will use for the first workout. So, if you can do 3 perfect bicep curls with 20-pound weights, then use 10-pound weights for your workout. Using this quick, efficient method before every new workout will help you determine how much weight to use. Some people will start with 2-pound weights, others will require 12 or 20 pounds. Once you're able to complete 5 or more circuits you'll then increase the weight.

Choose *1* exercise from each category below for a total of 4 exercises for each workout. Perform one set of 12 repetitions for each exercise followed immediately by the next exercise, stopping to rest any time you need to (within a set or between sets) and then starting right where you left off when you are ready. Each exercise features two movements, resulting in what we call hybrid exercises. For instance, a "squat/curl" means that you do arm curls with a dumbbell in each hand and squat each time you curl the dumbbells up toward your shoulders. Each group of exercises goes from easiest to most difficult.

Before starting the workout, warm up by completing several rounds of the hybrid exercises without weights as described below. At the end of your workout, cool down for 5 minutes by stretching all of your major muscle groups, including your neck.

SHOULD YOU WORK OUT ON AN EMPTY STOMACH?

The question of whether you should work out on an empty stomach is a controversial topic in the fitness world. Athletes who want to improve their performances have to eat before a workout so they have enough energy to push harder and further. But when it comes to exercising for fat loss, there are several considerations. First, you want to burn as many calories as possible during the time you exercise. Next, you want to work out in a way that creates the proper hormone balance to ensure maximal fat usage. Third, you want to try to maximize the metabolic effect (known in exercise science as EPOC), the afterburn created from intense exercise. Exercising first thing in the morning on an empty stomach provides benefits in two out of the three points above and may, depending on the individual, enhance all three. Studies show that workouts on an empty stomach burn more fat than those when food was eaten a few hours prior to the workout.

Many people just don't feel well when they exercise on an empty stomach and their workout quality will suffer. So despite all the science and logical arguments regarding eating and exercise, it ultimately comes back to common sense. The best advice is to do whatever allows you to generate the most intensity in your workouts and be consistent. If you are someone who is able to generate significant workout intensity without eating, then do so. If your workout quality suffers when you don't eat, then eat. Ultimately your results will be determined by how consistent you are with exercise, not by whether you eat or not before a workout.

If you don't do well exercising on an empty stomach and want to maximize your calorie usage, fat burning, and hormonal afterburn, here is a tip: Eat protein before a workout. Dissolve a scoop of whey protein in 8 ounces of water and drink it 30 to 45 minutes before a workout.

REST-BASED TRAINING (RBT)

The ME Workouts use a unique approach we developed called Rest-Based Training (RBT). This involves periods of intense exertion followed by voluntary rest. Unlike traditional workouts where rest is defined or always taken between exercises, Rest-Based Training allows you, the exerciser, to control when you rest and for how long. With Rest-Based Training you can pause either while exercising or between sets. There is no defined number of sets to complete in a workout— just complete as much work as possible within the allowed time. The Metabolic Exertion Scale (see page 75) is the major feedback tool in Rest-Based Training, allowing you to know when to rest and when to proceed. With Rest-Based Training you are competing with no one but yourself, so you should rest as often and for as long as is required; that way you can push hard when you start again. Some people take lots of short rests lasting only 10 to 20 seconds, while others take fewer rests lasting several minutes.

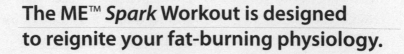

The ME™ *Spark* Workout is designed to reignite your fat-burning physiology.

① 12 reps,
then next

② 12 reps,
then next

③ 12 reps,
then next

④ 12 reps,
then start
again

20 minutes

Do 12 reps of each exercise in a
continuous circuit

Rest when needed

5 Workout Rules:

✔ **Choose 4** hybrid exercises.

✔ Do each exercise **12 times** &
immediately start the next exercise.

✔ Do a circuit repeating each exercise
one right after the other.

✔ **Rest** when you need to—then…
start again right where you left off.

✔ Complete as many rounds as
possible in **20 minutes.**

After picking the correct weights (see
below), follow the 5 workout rules listed.
Attempt to complete at least 4 rounds in
20 minutes with a goal of 5 rounds. After
you are able to get through 5 rounds,
increase your weight by 2.5–5 pounds in
each dumbbell. Once you choose your
workout do it 6 times over a 2-week
period before choosing a new workout
with 4 different exercises.

Guide to Choosing Weights:
Do 3 perfect dumbbell bicep curls
(not 2, not 4, but 3), then cut the amount
of weight in half. Use this weight to start
each new workout.

WARMING UP AND COOLING DOWN

While many people think they should stretch before a workout, research shows it's not as beneficial as preparing the body with a lighter version of the same activity you are about to do. Stretching should be done at the end of a workout, not the beginning.

Once you decide which hybrid exercises you're going to do, warm up by doing 1 to 3 rounds of the same exercises but without any weights. This is called a dynamic warm-up. Do each exercise 12 times, using a deliberate and slow full range of motion, working to feel the light stretches and contractions induced by the exercises. Once you feel "warm" or 5 minutes have passed, it's time to start the workout.

Set your timer for 20 minutes and, using weights, work as hard as you can until you have to rest (reaching a 4 on the Metabolic Exertion Scale). Then rest completely and resume the workout when you are back at a 1 or 2 on the Metabolic Exertion Scale.

After completing your workout, walk slowly for a minute or two, allowing your heart rate to come down. Then stretch all the major muscle groups: the front and back of the legs, the chest and the back and the neck. Hold each stretch for ten seconds or longer. Do not bounce while stretching.

The best way to avoid injury and get the most out of your workout is to warm up for 2 to 5 minutes before working out and stretch for 5 minutes to cool down. Your body and your metabolism will perform at their best if allowed to ease into and out of the process.

THE METABOLIC EXERTION SCALE

As stated previously, use the 1 to 4 rating scale called the Metabolic Exertion Scale to determine how to tailor your workout to your individual fitness level. Here's a reminder:

1. You are at rest and are not exerting yourself.

2. Exercise is easy. You can still talk. You feel no burn in your muscles and/or the weight feels easy to lift.

3. You are working out hard. You are no longer able to talk. Your muscles are burning and/or the weight is very heavy. You are starting to generate a metabolic effect!

4. You can no longer continue to exercise. You experience severe muscle burn and/or the weights feel too heavy. You have to rest. At this phase, there is a dramatic increase in the muscle-building, fat-burning hormones. This number 4 stage is what we call the Metabolic Effect Point.

Heart-Rate Monitors

Many people like to wear heart-rate monitors while working out to assess workout intensity and maintain safety. The ME Workouts use heart-rate monitors differently. Many believe in the "fat-burning zone," an area usually described as between 65 to 80 percent maximum heart rate. This is where you are supposed to burn the highest proportion of fat. But you have already learned that the real fat-burning zone occurs when the body is pushed above the aerobic zone, which for most people occurs when the maximum heart rate is above 85 percent. If you can breach 85 percent maximum heart rate multiple times in a workout, you are achieving the metabolic effect. If you don't have a heart-rate monitor, use the Metabolic Exertion Scale (page 75) to monitor intensity. If you prefer the additional feedback of a heart-rate monitor, here are the numbers to know.

220 – your age = Max Heart Rate (MHR)
MHR × .85 = 85% MHR
MHR × .72 = 72% MHR

Let's say you're a 40-year-old woman:
220 – 40 = 180
180 × .85 = 153
180 × .72 = 130

With a heart-rate monitor the goal is to maintain 72 percent during ME Workouts, which corresponds to a 2 on the metabolic exertion scale. Every few minutes spike your heart rate up to 85 percent MHR or more for brief periods, and then come back down to 72 percent. (You will see the beats per minute on your monitor.) Let's say that you spike to more than 85 percent on your monitor and that you're able to maintain that for 30 seconds before resting. When you rest, before your heart rate begins to drop, it will jump a few more beats and then proceed to fall again. As an example, if you sprint for 1 minute and then rest, for the first 10 seconds of your resting period your heart rate will actually go up, an indication that you successfully created an EPOC effect/metabolic effect. Remember that certain drugs and illnesses can impact the response of the heart. If you have any medical concerns or issues, you should speak with your physician before attempting any type of exercise regimen. Heart-rate recovery (HRR) is a sensitive indicator of your heart health. An optimally healthy heart should be able to recover at least 20 beats per minute with rest after exertion.

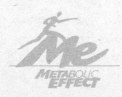

WALKING: YOUR SYNERGISTIC FAT BURNER

In addition to the 30-minute intense workouts, you should walk every day for at least 30 to 60 minutes. We suggest walking for 30 minutes on the days you do your rest-based workouts and 30 to 60 minutes on off days. At the very least, walk on the days you don't do your rest-based workouts. Walking acts as a synergistic fat burner when combined with the rest-based more intense ME Workouts.

Walking should not be seen as exercise but rather as a necessity. Your ancestors walked all day every day. Walking is a magical exercise because it regulates your hormonal stress response in a positive way. Walking lowers stress hormones, sensitizes insulin, and ensures a constant and steady release of the metabolic messengers. Walking and higher-intensity activities like intense weight lifting, interval training, or sprinting work in a synergistic fashion to regulate the metabolism. They act as the yin and yang of exercise. Walking is yin, or calming, while the ME Workouts are yang, or stimulating. The other type of exercise, intense lifting and sprinting, activates the stimulating side of the nervous system and creates growth and a metabolic fat-burning burst. The high-intensity activity assures that the calories you burn while you walk are fat and not sugar. Combined with the high-intensity workouts, walking guarantees that stress hormones/growth hormone balance is in favor of growth. Other types of exercise that work synergistically with the ME Workout include restorative yoga, tai chi, and qi gong.

Whether you walk outdoors or on a treadmill, your pace should be brisk. You should be at a 2 on the Metabolic Exertion Scale (page 75). This means that you are exerting yourself but you can still carry on a conversation with someone.

Some people like to use a pedometer, which tells them exactly how many steps they take. Aim for 5,000 to 10,000 paces daily, or whatever you can achieve in 30 to 60 minutes.

What about traditional cardiovascular exercises like jogging, running, biking, or using an elliptical trainer? Many experts and fitness enthusiasts still push this "aerobic zone" type of exercise as the only form of exercise needed. Again, they're operating from the world of weight loss, not fat loss. Aerobic zone exercise is not as beneficial as walking and high-intensity exercise because it can't generate the same hormonal effect. Like walking, aerobic exercise burns calories but creates little afterburn, so while you may be using energy for the hour you're exercising, once you stop, so does fat burning. While walking decreases stress hormones relative to growth hormones, aerobic exercise pushes the equation more toward the stress side.

Like high-intensity exercise, the longer you do this activity the more stress hormones you produce, but unlike high-intensity exercise there are no growth hormones triggered to turn the stress hormones into fat-burning allies. Remember the differences between elite sprinters and top-level marathon runners. They are both lean, but sprinters often have less body fat, more muscle, and a much healthier appearance.

What about other sports and physical activities? Whether you play basketball, swim laps, cycle, hike, or take yoga or Pilates instruction, know that all exercise is good for you, but to reap fat-burning and muscle-building benefits, there's no substitute for intense rest-based exercise combined with low-intensity walking.

○   ○   ○

Optimal Metabolic Rest-Based Intervals

Many people can't find the time to walk every day or want to do more to elevate their fat-burning potential. That is where ME rest-based interval training can be useful. Interval training is a system of exercise in which periods of intense activity are followed by periods of slow, active rest. The problem is, the work intervals and periods of rest can be too long for many, too short for others. Rest-based intervals are short, just 30 minutes including a warm-up and a cool-down period, and can be done in between the rest-based weight-training circuit workouts. Here's how:

- Complete a 5-minute warm-up staying at a 2 on the Metabolic Exertion Scale.
- Do sets of the following: a 20-second sprint, followed by as much rest as you require; then a 30-second sprint, followed by rest until you are ready to go again; then a 40-second sprint, followed by more rest. Finally, when you are ready, a 1-minute sprint, followed by rest according to your needs. Repeat the entire circuit, completing as many rounds as possible in 20 minutes.
- Cool down by slowly walking or pedaling a stationary bike or elliptical trainer at a metabolic exertion of 2 for 5 minutes and the workout is done.

During the sprints, your metabolic exertion should be at 3 throughout, reaching 4 when the sprint is finished. Rest for the appropriate time and go again. During the rest periods, walk or pedal in almost slow motion while you take deep breaths to recover. These workouts can be done by all fitness levels and can take the place of walking workouts. A good mix of the ME weight-training workouts, these metabolic intervals, and walking works best.

Remember, walking can be done anytime, anywhere. You can never walk too much! Here's a suggested workout schedule using weight training, metabolic intervals, and walking:

Monday:	metabolic rest-based circuit and 30-minute walk
Tuesday:	30-minute metabolic intervals
Wednesday:	metabolic rest-based circuit and 30-minute walk
Thursday:	30-minute metabolic intervals
Friday:	metabolic rest-based circuit and 30-minute walk
Saturday:	30- to 60-minute walk
Sunday:	30- to 60-minute walk

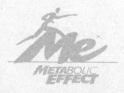

KNOWING WHEN THE METABOLIC SPARK IS WORKING AND WHEN YOU ARE READY FOR STAGE II: THE METABOLIC TRANSFORMATION

For those with an already healthy metabolism, in 7 days you'll not only feel better, but your face will look thinner. You will see new contours in your shape. You will also experience a 5- to 15-pound weight loss depending on what kind of burner you are. This is usually more dramatic in sugar burners. This weight loss is water weight, which signals that you have sparked your metabolism and that your metabolism has switched to burning fat. You are now ready to move into the fast lane of the Metabolic Spark and for the first few months you will burn 0.5 to 1 percent body fat per week and add metabolic muscle.

For others, it may take up to 10 days to feel better and from 1 to 4 weeks to see a loss of water weight. Some people have headaches due to the lower blood sugar that can occur during this period. Close adherence to your nutrition by adjusting the proportion of protein, fiber, and starch according to your metabolic plate will easily remedy this.

In general, experience has shown us that people feel great within a week, have increased energy, and sleep better.

Creating a Metabolic Spark may have occurred fairly quickly for you, or it may have taken some time. Everyone is different and responds uniquely to changes in diet, exercise, and lifestyle. Most people will find that they can complete the Spark Stage of the program and make the switch into the fat-burning and muscle-building Transformation Stage in 3 weeks to 3 months. To fully benefit from the hormonal changes taking place at this time, it is best to continue the Spark Stage for the full 3 months. Some people, such as former athletes, can see this shift in their metabolism in as little as 3 days, though this is rare. In order to achieve a large enough Metabolic Spark to ignite your fat-burning potential, diet is extremely important and accounts for about 75 percent of your success during this phase. It takes an awareness of what you're eating and adjusting your diet to get it right.

You may feel shifts in your physiology, which indicate changes in blood sugar. These might include headaches, brief disruptions in sleep, or lows in energy in the morning or afternoon. These occurrences mean that you have effectively lowered the amount of sugar available to the body for energy, but that the body hasn't yet picked up the slack with adequate fat burning. It's important in the Spark Stage to remember that you can quickly and frequently slip out of fat-burning mode. Those "symptoms" are valuable tools when it comes to knowing how to manage fat burning. Pay close attention to how frequently you eat, consume adequate protein and fiber, and adjust your bites of starch. The biofeedback tools of hunger, energy, and cravings will be useful guides to your progress as you move into the transformation part of the program.

BACK HYBRIDS (choose one)

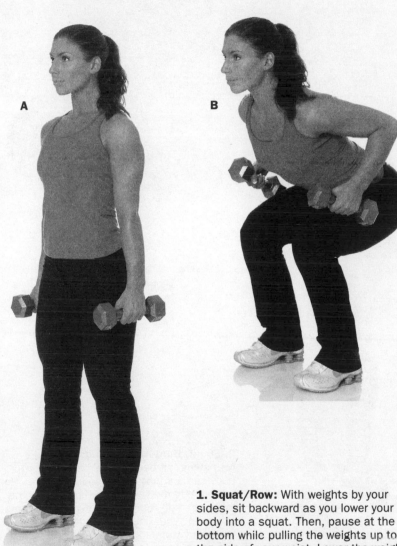

1. Squat/Row: With weights by your sides, sit backward as you lower your body into a squat. Then, pause at the bottom while pulling the weights up to the side of your waist. Lower the weights and return to standing. Repeat 12 times.

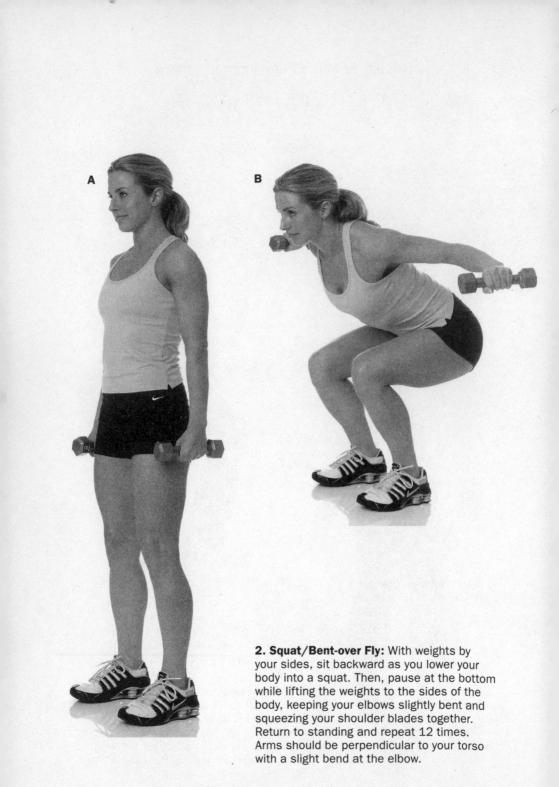

2. Squat/Bent-over Fly: With weights by your sides, sit backward as you lower your body into a squat. Then, pause at the bottom while lifting the weights to the sides of the body, keeping your elbows slightly bent and squeezing your shoulder blades together. Return to standing and repeat 12 times. Arms should be perpendicular to your torso with a slight bend at the elbow.

A

B

C

3. Static Squat/Row/Fly:
With weights by your sides,
hold yourself in a squatting
position with your weights
hanging just in front of your
knees. Then pull the weights
straight up and even with
your waist. Lower them and
bring them out to the sides
with your arms perpendicular
to your torso, keeping your
elbows slightly bent. Repeat
these two movements in a
continuous motion 12 times.

A

4. In Place Lunge/Row: Standing with your feet together and holding dumbbells by your sides, take a big step forward with your right leg and drop your back knee straight down toward the ground. Your front knee should fall in line with your front ankle, creating a 90-degree angle between your upper and lower leg. Lean forward at the waist and pull the weights up by squeezing your shoulder blades together and bending your arms. The weights should be even with your belly button. Relax the arms and then push back forcefully on the front heel to return to a standing position before repeating the movement on the other side. Do 6 repetitions on each leg for 12 rows total.

B

CHEST HYBRIDS (choose one)

A

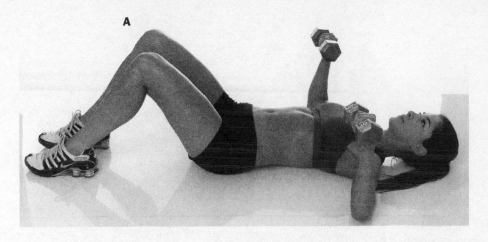

1. Chest Press/Crunch: Lying on your back, press the weights up toward the ceiling while lifting your shoulder blades off the floor and contracting your abs. Hold this position for a count of 2, release, and repeat 12 times.

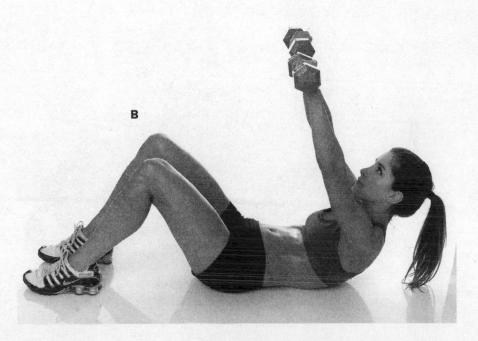

B

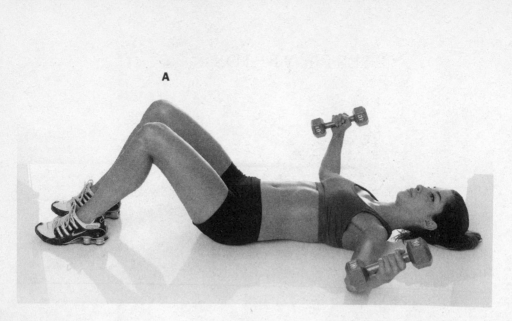

A

2. Chest Fly/Crunch: Lying on your back, bring the weights out toward the sides of the body in an arcing motion until they meet in front of you with arms slightly bent and dumbbells touching. Squeeze the weights together, as if you are giving someone a hug, and lift your shoulder blades off the floor at the same time and contract your abs. Hold this position for a count of 2, release, and repeat 12 times.

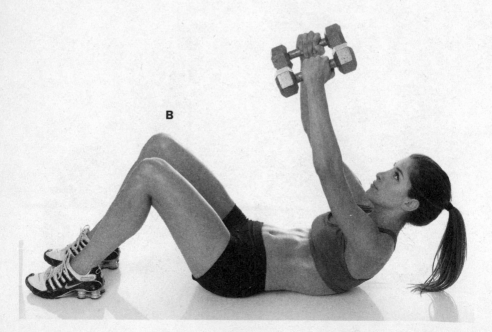

B

A

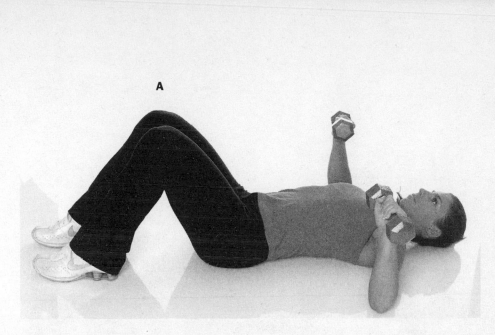

3. Chest Press/Chest Fly: Lying on your back, press the weights straight up toward the ceiling, then slowly lower the weights by bending the elbows slightly and, in a wide arcing pattern, let the arms move out to the sides of the body. Bring the weights back up in the same arcing pattern (fly). When the weights are at the top, lower them straight down. Repeat the entire movement 12 times.

B

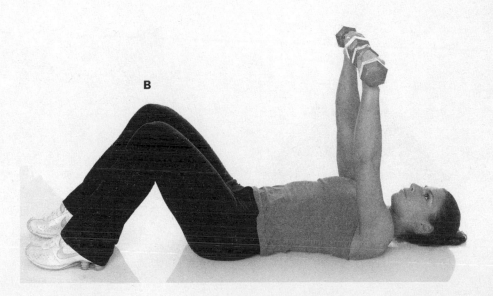

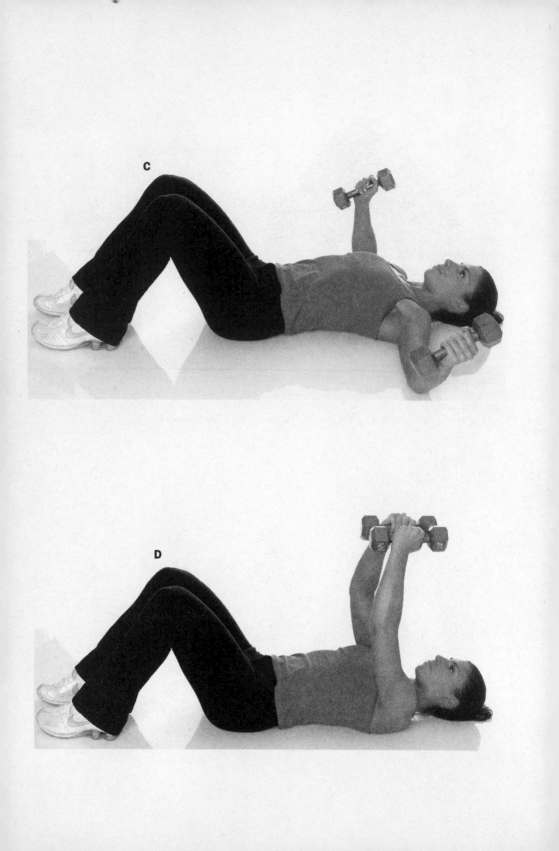

A

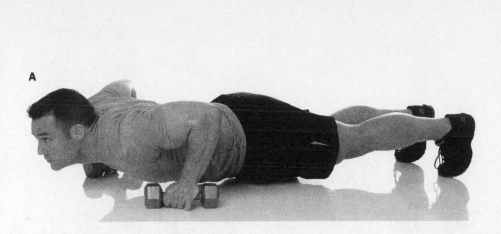

4. Push-up/Row: In a push-up position (on the knees or the toes) with the dumbbells in your hands, do a push-up by lowering your chest toward the floor. As you push back up, row one weight to the side of the body. Lower that weight and repeat the push-up, then row the other weight. Continue alternating, doing a push-up and a row on one side followed by a push-up and then a row on the other side for a total of 12 repetitions.

B

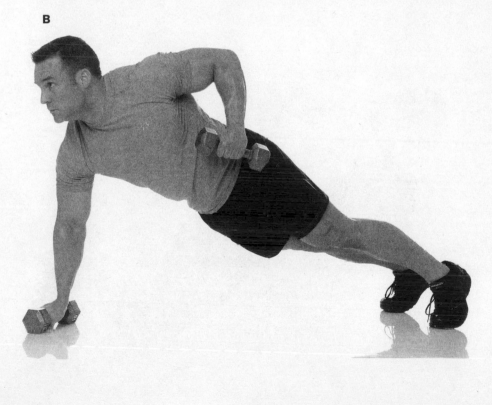

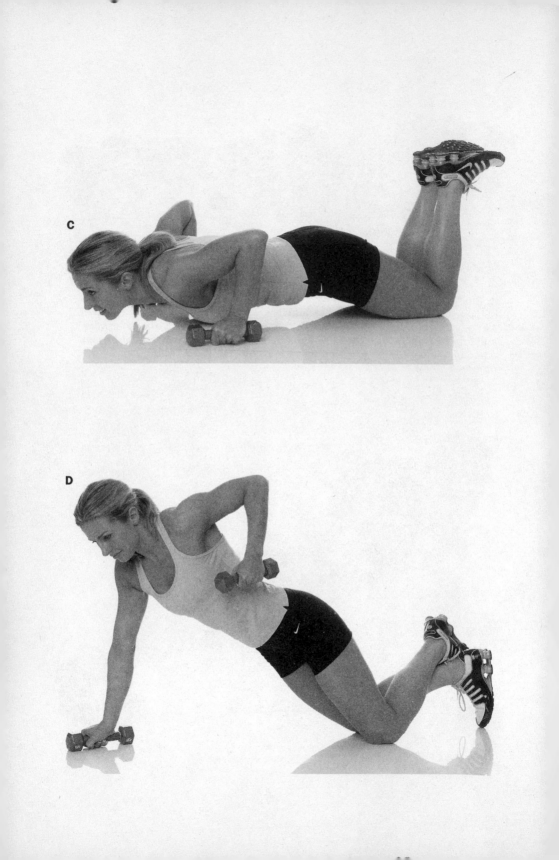

ARM HYBRIDS (choose one)

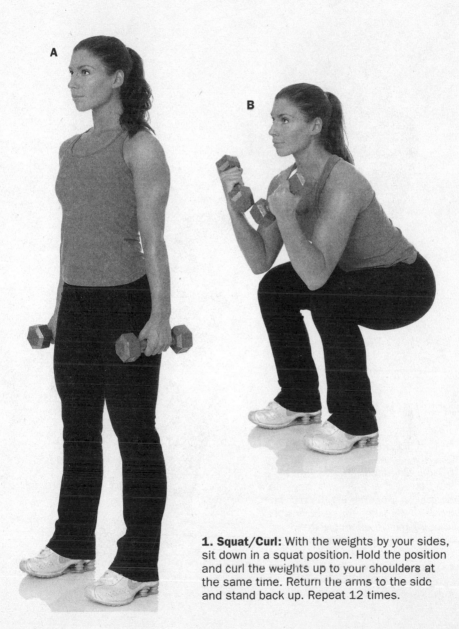

1. Squat/Curl: With the weights by your sides, sit down in a squat position. Hold the position and curl the weights up to your shoulders at the same time. Return the arms to the side and stand back up. Repeat 12 times.

A

B

2. Curl/Extension: Holding yourself in a squat position with the weights by your sides, curl the weights to the front of the body, and then in a controlled motion bring the elbows close to the sides of the body while keeping the arms bent. Extend the arms up and back into a tricep extension. Repeat the movement by alternating between the curl and extension 12 times, staying in a squat position throughout.

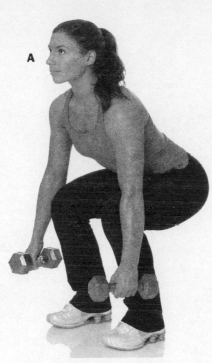

A

B

C

3. Row/Extension: In a squat position, let the weights hang straight down. Pull the weights up to the waist while squeezing the shoulder blades. Without taking tension off the shoulder blades, straighten the elbows so that the weights are behind the body in a tricep extension. Reverse. Repeat the entire movement 12 times.

A

B

C

4. Lunge/Curl/Press: Step into a lunge position and curl the weights from the sides of the body to shoulder level, then press the weights straight overhead. Lower the weights to your sides and push back to a standing position. Lunge on the other side and repeat the entire movement 12 times (6 lunges on each leg and 12 curl/press).

SHOULDER HYBRIDS (choose one)

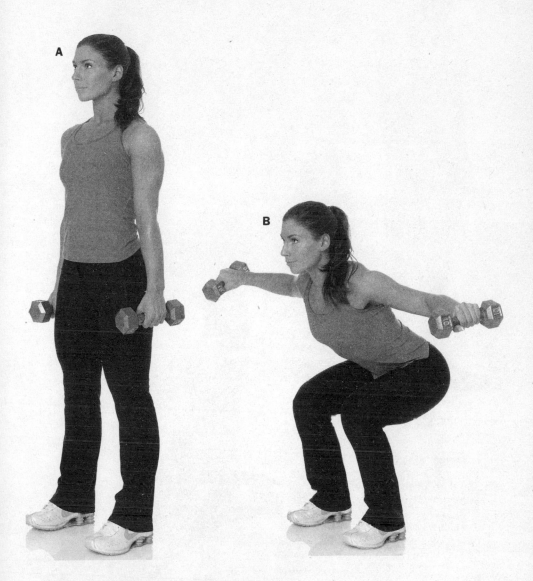

1. Squat/Side Raise: Squat down, then lift the weights out to the sides of the body, keeping the elbows slightly bent. Then bring the arms back down, stand back up, and repeat the movement 12 times.

A

B

2. Lunge/Side Raise:
Step into a lunge position and then lift the weights straight out to the sides of the body, keeping the elbows bent and not lifting past shoulder height. Bring the arms down to the sides of the body. Push back to standing and repeat on the opposite side. Repeat this entire movement 12 times (6 lunges on each leg and 12 side raises).

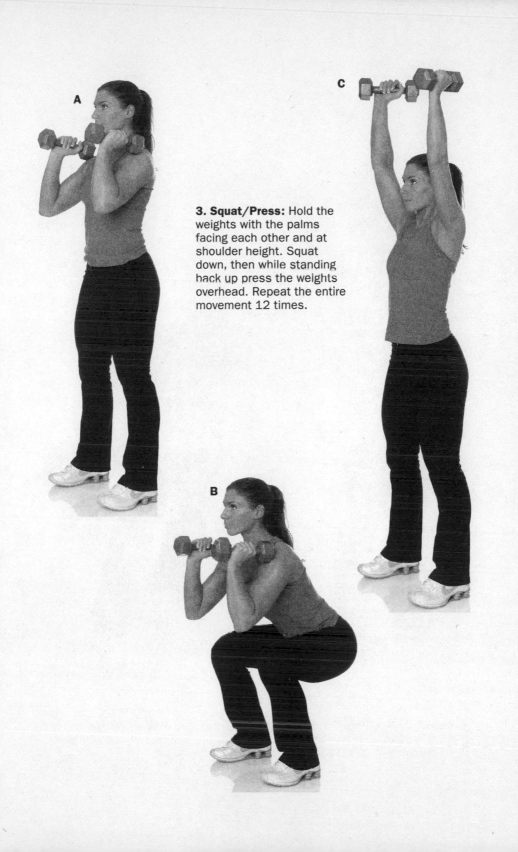

3. Squat/Press: Hold the weights with the palms facing each other and at shoulder height. Squat down, then while standing back up press the weights overhead. Repeat the entire movement 12 times.

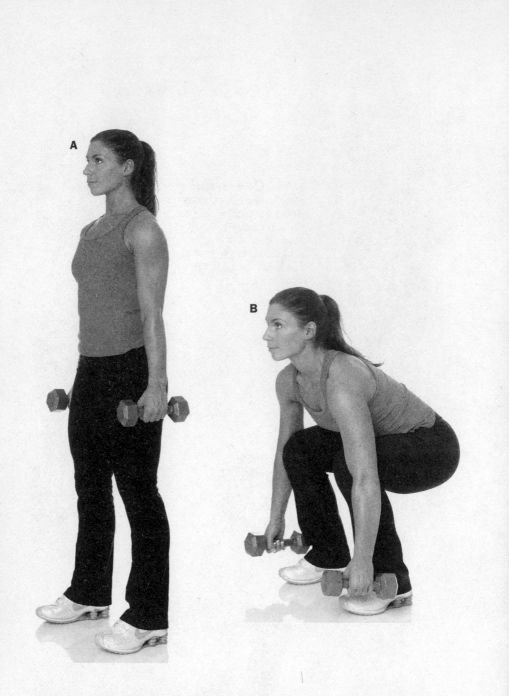

4. Dead Lift/Curl/Press: With the weights by the sides of your body, squat until the weights touch the ground. As you stand up, curl the weights, then press them overhead. Repeat 12 times.

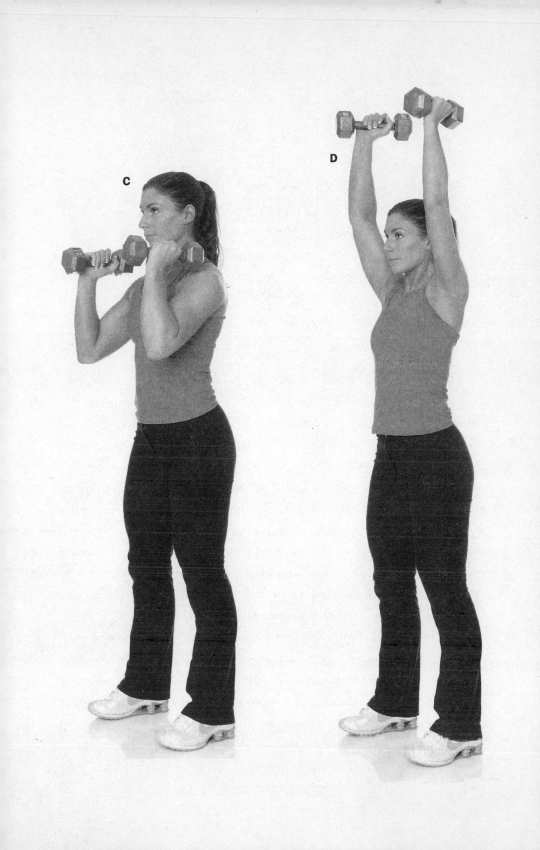

CHAPTER FIVE

THE METABOLIC TRANSFORMATION

The Metabolic Spark helped you reawaken your body's fat-burning potential by using food and exercise to trigger specific fat-burning hormones. Now your body is beginning to fire on all cylinders and has the information on whether to burn or store fat and is responding by releasing metabolic messengers.

The goal of the Metabolic Transformation is to make a lasting change from a metabolism that runs primarily on sugar to one that consistently burns fat. Remember, your metabolism can supply its sugar-burning needs through stored sugar (glycogen) from food or by breaking down muscle tissue and using those amino acids to make sugar. In order to permanently retrain the metabolism to burn fat, you need to learn how to harness the power of your muscles in new ways.

During the Metabolic Spark Stage we focused mainly on the indirect effects diet and exercise have on hormone signaling by employing a high-intensity workout that combines elements of both resistance training and interval exercise. As a result, you were able to manipulate the adrenal glands (stress glands) to release metabolic messengers to generate an elevated fat-burning metabolism for days. In the Metabolic Transformation Stage, you'll focus on building more muscle to take advantage of specific metabolic messengers called myokines. These are metabolic messengers released directly by the muscle, as opposed to the indirect effect generated from the adrenal burst of hormones.

The concept that muscles send signals into the body is confusing to many people because we are so conditioned to think of our muscles as simply our "locomotion anatomy" that allows us to move. While that's true, muscles are also a powerful source of myokines. The amount of muscle mass on your body and how you move those muscles sends metabolic messages directly to the brain, liver, and fat cells regulating how much you eat, how much fat you burn, and how much muscle you continue to build.

The number of these specific muscle molecules depends on several factors: how much energy muscles have stored as sugar, how much muscle is being moved, and how intensely the muscle is being moved or exercised. And, the more muscle you have, the more beneficial the response. You learned in the Metabolic Spark Stage how hybrid exercises work many different muscle groups at the same time. In the Metabolic Transformation Workout two key elements are added to enhance the number of muscle molecules you release and to help maintain or even gain valuable muscle: an increase in the amount of weight lifted and the degree of muscle burn.

The only way to guarantee that your body will burn fat at rest is to build muscle. People with a higher percentage of muscle mass have an advantage in relearning how to burn fat after a period of weight gain.

The negative results and the impact of low-calorie, aerobic-exercise diets have been known for many years in the scientific community. A study published in the *Journal of the American College of Nutrition* (April 1999) showed just how effective muscle is at maintaining metabolic potential. Obese people were put on a very low-calorie diet, with one group doing aerobic exercise (walking, biking, or jogging 4 times per week) and another group doing resistance exercise 3 times per week. At the end of the 12-week study, both groups had lost weight, but the difference in the type of weight lost was striking. The aerobic group lost

28 pounds of fat and 9 pounds of muscle. The resistance-training group lost 32 pounds of fat and little to no muscle. When the resting metabolic rate of each group was calculated at the end of the study, the aerobic group had a huge reduction in energy usage at rest, decreasing their resting calorie usage by 210 calories per day. In contrast, the resistance-training group increased their metabolisms by 63 calories per day.

HOW YOU KNOW THE METABOLIC SPARK IS WORKING AND THAT YOU'RE READY FOR THE METABOLIC TRANSFORMATION STAGE

The first sign that you are moving from the Metabolic Spark Stage to the Metabolic Transformation Stage will be a redistribution or loss of water weight. Many fat-storing hormones also indirectly affect how the body stores water. This is often seen in the subcutaneous (under the skin) areas. You (and perhaps others) will notice that your face and the area around your middle are smaller or thinner. The waistband on your clothes will be looser by ½ to 1 inch. Friends may ask, "Have you lost weight?" You will experience a drop in weight from a few pounds to 10 or more. Almost all the weight lost is water weight, but it is a direct indication that you have entered fat-burning mode. As you shift into a more consistent fat-burning state, you will experience increased vitality. Most people describe this phase as feeling that a fog has been lifted off them. They feel lighter, more motivated, and notice that they have more endurance and greater energy. Their workouts become easier; there's less soreness and a faster recovery.

For some people, the loss of water at this point isn't as dramatic. Don't despair. First, remember that sugar burners, who are usually overweight, lose the most water at this stage. Second, make sure you're drinking enough water. Third, cut back on the amount of salt in your diet. Too much salt affects fat loss, causing you to retain excess water and to have a puffy or bloated look. Salt also interrupts the natural cycle of nervous-system function, leading to unfavorable changes in fat-burning hormones. Our bodies were developed over the millennia to consume about 700mg of sodium and 11,000mg of potassium per day, but each day the average American consumes 4,000mg or more of sodium and 4,000mg or less of potassium. The sodium-potassium ratio is a crucial part of a fat-burning diet. As sodium levels rise in relation to potassium levels, the internal pH of a cell becomes more acidic, interrupting the ability of fat-burning enzymes to do their job effectively. Unless this ratio is reversed, cellular fat burning becomes almost impossible. The body does a good job in regulating this ratio to keep itself functioning, but to ensure that you make the transformation into a fat-burning state, cut back on your salt intake by not adding salt to your food and avoiding excessively salty meals. Increasing the amount of vegetables and fruit you eat and eliminating salt will restore the sodium-potassium ratio and get you burning fat again. Ironically, many of the fat-storing hormones like insulin and cortisol lead to sodium retention. Reducing production of these hormones and inducing a better sodium-potassium ratio are powerful one-two punches that will help restore your fat-burning metabolism.

MUSCLES TALK

Muscles are huge reservoirs of metabolic signaling. Every time you move, you release metabolic messengers from muscle cells that "speak" directly to the liver, fat cells, and brain, impacting every aspect of your body's metabolism. So, the more muscle—and less fat—you have, the greater the body's capacity to reengineer its metabolism, which is why the ME program works. Since aerobic exercise burns rather than builds muscle, it fails to deliver a metabolic change that is sustainable.

Muscles "talk" to the rest of the body during exercise and add to the favorable hormonal changes the body is exposed to, which causes enhanced fat burning. These muscle molecules also impact the release of muscle-building hormones like growth hormone and testosterone to increase muscle mass, creating a simultaneous muscle-building and fat-burning effect.

The amount of muscle hormones released is directly related to how many muscles are moved during exercise and how fatigued the muscles become. This is why the ME program uses combination exercises (hybrids) that employ the entire body and why a rest-based workout regimen is key to burning fat. The old method of doing a few repetitions of an exercise and then resting without reaching the point of full fatigue doesn't generate the same muscle molecule response and therefore is a less effective form of exercise. Using more muscle mass, combining cardiovascular exercise with resistance training, and training until you are exhausted and must rest significantly ignites a fat-burning fire that can last for days! These exercises create a stimulus strong enough to generate the release of testosterone and growth hormone, which are able to aid fat loss, but more important, turn the body's muscle-making machinery back on. These two hormones are potent stimulators for the development of new muscle tissue.

ADD MUSCLE, BURN FAT

In the Metabolic Transformation, the goal is to make a permanent transition from a metabolism that runs primarily on sugar to one that consistently burns fat. This process is about retaining the hormonal changes you made in the Spark Stage and ensuring that they last. Keeping fat off the body involves not only burning fat, but building muscle too. It is important to understand that a reduction in muscle mass is disastrous to a fat-burning metabolism. Muscle is key to your fat-burning physiology, yet this is a concept that is ignored by every major weight-loss program, fad diet, or major study done on body composition. You cannot transform your body without sculpting new muscle mass.

HOW TO MEASURE FAT LOSS VERSUS MUSCLE LOSS

Knowing how much fat you are losing is entirely different from measuring your weight. Traditional scales only measure pounds lost, not the amount of muscle or fat, which is why you should invest in a body-fat scale. This simple device measures the amount of fat versus muscle you are losing, allowing you to be completely aware of your transformation. We use and recommend Tanita brand.

Obviously, if you are losing more muscle than fat, you are not making a transformation at all, but, rather, are disrupting your metabolic efficiency. You also want to be aware of how a loss in water will affect your body-fat percentage. During the transition from the Metabolic Spark to the consistent and sustained Metabolic Transformation, you will lose water. While water loss is a beneficial biofeedback tool that signals the reduction in fat-storing hormones, it is often a point of confusion when using body-fat scales. These devices read a loss in water as muscle loss, since water is present to a much larger degree in muscle than it is in fat. This, in turn, elevates the percent of body fat the machine registers. This response is only an issue during the first few weeks of the ME fat-burning diet. Don't be confused if you see your body-fat percent artificially rise due to this "water effect" before it consistently begins to drop. Being aware of the metabolic process in your body and how these scales work allows you to monitor your progress efficiently and avoid weight-loss diets that decrease metabolic efficiency.

THE BENEFITS OF MUSCLES: LOOK GOOD, FEEL GOOD, LIVE LONGER

Many people, women in particular, are afraid of building muscle mass. To them it conjures up images of freakishly muscled men and women hoisting barbells over their heads in bodybuilding contests. Think about your favorite top-level athletes—tennis players, swimmers, and basketball players of either gender. They don't look bulky or freakish, do they? They look lean, sculpted, and fit. That's because proper athletic conditioning allows them to lose fat yet maintain and add muscle mass. The muscles you develop with the ME Workout create that much admired and desired lean but fit look.

Muscles, fat, and other types of tissues differ from one another in many ways. Muscles are metabolically active and use a tremendous amount of energy when moving and at rest. In fact, muscles burn up to 2 to 10 times more calories while at rest than fat or other tissue. Fat and other body tissues are much more inert when resting, more like a storage depot where energy is housed. For every pound of muscle you gain, you will burn an additional 6 to 30 calories per day by doing nothing. But here's the really good part: the more muscle you have on your frame, the more your fat-burning potential increases once a workout is finished, and it can last for up to 48 hours afterward.

Don't be disappointed when you step on the scale in the early days and weeks of the ME program and don't see the pounds dropping immediately. Your weight on a traditional scale may not change very much despite the loss of significant amounts of fat. A pound of muscle and a pound of fat each weigh the same amount, but muscle is denser than fat, which means that it takes up less space on your body. If you are putting on muscle and burning fat, your body-fat percentage will decrease, but your weight won't drop considerably at this point. This means the body will not only shrink in size, but will also improve its shape and tone, another major difference between fat loss and weight loss. When the focus is only on weight loss, your body may get smaller, but its shape won't change. If you're pear shaped, you'll become a smaller pear shape, and we've all seen people who've lost a lot of weight, only to find that their skin becomes loose and saggy.

A fat-burning body becomes smaller *and* the shape of the body changes. Muscle tissue, unlike fat tissue, can drastically change both the size, tone, and shape of the body, pulling connective tissue and skin closer to the body and minimizing saggy areas. As a result, the body not only looks firmer, it actually is firmer. As you burn fat and build muscle with the ME Diet, you'll drop inches, your clothes will be looser, and your face will look thinner.

The benefits of muscles go beyond looking and feeling good. Think of muscles as a built-in antiaging delivery system. The same muscles that release hormones to burn fat and assist in gaining muscle mass also decrease inflammation throughout the body and have a positive antiaging effect. Toned and fit muscles spur the body to make more muscles. The actual tugging on bones against gravity when muscles move induces bone growth.

Barbara: An Individual Approach

When Barbara came to us, she was desperate. "My daughters are 9, 7, and almost 5. I was fit most of my life, until having children. I had three children in 4½ years, so that pretty much wrecked my body. I gained weight after each child and never lost it."

Thirty-four-year-old Barbara was almost 100 pounds overweight. She wanted to lose the weight, but was clearly having trouble finding the time and the motivation to work out. Three daughters didn't leave Barbara with much time for herself. What was especially frustrating to Barbara was that until she started having children she had been fit all of her life.

Her old ways of staying thin and fit—eat less, exercise more—no longer worked. Her willpower was constantly challenged and her schedule was never her own. When we met with her, she said, "I want to feel better. I know if I could lose weight, I'd have more energy. But it seems that I just don't have time for me."

After determining that she was a mixed burner, we suggested that Barbara join one of our outdoor group workouts at a regularly scheduled time 3 to 5 times a week while her girls were in school. She was surprised by how much she could accomplish in a 30-minute workout. The more she rested, the harder she pushed.

As a mixed burner, her new diet allowed her to eat 6 times a day. At major meals she was allowed 10 or fewer bites of starch. Like all of our clients, Barbara was instructed on how to use hunger, cravings, and energy to guide her diet and the amount of protein, fiber, and starch she ate. She discovered that her new diet wasn't one of deprivation and that it worked with her schedule (eating frequent meals and snacks, like her kids).

During the first 8 weeks of diet and exercise she lost more than 5 percent of her body fat. Her body's shape began to change and her focus switched from weight loss to fat loss. After 9 months Barbara had lost 89 pounds and her body fat had dropped from 40 percent to 20 percent.

What surprised Barbara and the rest of us is how athletic she has become and how much she now enjoys working out. She is one of the fastest sprinters in her group and usually finishes first. Barbara now has a small waist and muscular, not bulky, arms. Her skin is firm and taut. Most of all, Barbara has become an inspiration to her friends. When they ask her for advice, she tells them, "What I love about the ME Diet is that it isn't a one-size-fits-all program. Instead, the diet and workout are individualized to fit into my lifestyle.

"I'm back to the size I was in college, but my husband repeatedly tells me how much more toned and fit I am now. I've noticed the most difference in my arms—the change is remarkable, and I have noticed how much stronger I am and how much more energy I have than ever before."

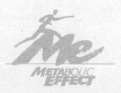

FOOD MESSENGERS

In the Spark Stage you discovered how important it is to integrate both diet and exercise for optimal fat loss. Just as we have switched to talking about the indirect versus the direct effects of exercise on muscle, the Transformation Stage of the ME Diet does the same with food and nutrition. In the Spark Stage you discovered that what you eat is information for the body and shouldn't be thought of as calories in, calories out. You now know that the foods you eat signal the release of specific hormones to turn fat burning on or off.

Certain foods contain compounds that speak directly to your metabolic machinery and your genes, sometimes bypassing your own hormonal software and acting as hormones themselves. We call these metabolic messengers "food messengers." These compounds, found in fruits, vegetables, and other foods, are called phytonutrients. They act as metabolic messengers by interacting with some of the same receptors our hormones do. These specific food messengers create a metabolic effect from the hormones released by your body, and some of these phytonutrients act as direct messenger molecules. These phytonutrients are found in many foods, including green tea, pomegranates, red wine, and chocolate. Certain fish and dairy products contain powerful fats that interact with cell receptors on the nucleus, turning fat-burning genes on. These fats work by binding to the receptors, called PPARs (peroxisome proliferator-activated receptors), present on the cell nucleus. When these receptors are activated, they send signals to the genes, turning some genes on and others off. Combining the indirect effects of food on hormones like insulin, glucagon, and leptin with the direct effects of food messengers on cell and nuclear receptors impacts your metabolic fat-burning potential with a potent one-two punch. You'll discover how eating these specific foods impacts one or both of these systems.

THE TRANSFORMATION DIET

During the Spark Stage you learned how to engineer your body's individual fat-burning mechanisms by eating certain foods and by monitoring your biofeedback tools of hunger, energy, and cravings. The specific food recommendations allowed you to transition into a steady fat-burning state. Follow the same diet you adhered to during the Spark Stage; it will continue to sustain your fat-loss efforts. You know how to use protein, fiber, starch, and fat to trigger your biochemistry to burn fat. In this chapter you'll be introduced to other foods and supplements that aid fat loss with specific recommendations for sugar, mixed, or muscle burners.

Certain fruits, vegetables, and fats act as these "food messengers." Other food additives like vinegar, natural sugar substitutes, and spices are valuable for their ability to adjust physiology in favor of fat burning. Based on what kind of burner you are, some of these foods may be more suitable than others, but they all provide benefits.

GOOD FATS

We know it seems odd to even suggest eating fat when this book is all about burning it. Again, you need to move away from thinking about calories. Looking at fat from a hormonal perspective allows you to shift your thinking to what messages fat might be sending. Most fats are hormonally neutral, but certain types act as metabolic messengers themselves. Two fats found in wild fish, game, and grass-fed beef have dramatic effects on fat burning. Called omega-3s, these fats are known as EPA (eicosapentenoic acid) and DHA (docosahexanoic acid). They act as metabolic messengers by directly interacting with receptors in cell membranes, resulting in an increased expression of genes that enhance fat metabolism. There is another type of fat derived from ruminant animals like cows called CLA (conjugated linoleic acid). Like

EPA and DHA, this fat is able to modulate genetic expression, resulting in shrinkage of the size and number of fat cells. CLA is found in high concentrations in milk fat, particularly milk derived from cattle that have been grass fed their entire lives. This remarkable food messenger can have substantial effects on fat burning.

Adding these fats to the diet can dramatically enhance your fat-burning potential. EPA and DHA can be made in the body, but because this system is slow in humans it takes almost 10g of oil from a rich plant source like flax to make just 1g of EPA or DHA. For this reason it is best to get these oils from wild, not farmed, fish. Canned salmon is a good source of these oils, because all canned salmon is processed from wild fish. Fresh, wild salmon is very expensive. In addition to salmon, smaller fish such as sardines, anchovies, herring, and mackerel are high in omega-3s and lowest in mercury content. Eat small amounts of big fish, such as tuna, halibut, or swordfish, which contain more mercury, infrequently.

Sources of these fats can also be found in flax and hemp oils and walnuts, which should be consumed in addition to fish. Vegetarians who don't eat fish should take 1 to 3 tablespoons of flax or hemp oil per day. Everyone benefits from sprinkling 2 tablespoons of flax meal on salads or their morning oatmeal.

WHEY PROTEIN POWDER

Whey protein powder, a dairy by-product, is a rich food source for developing muscles. Whey protein powder also aids in fat loss by lowering the stress hormone cortisol while raising the brain hormones dopamine and serotonin. Whey protein helps fight cravings, satisfies hunger hormones, boosts immunity, and stabilizes blood sugar. All of these positives, along with its powerful muscle-building ability, make it the ideal food for balancing your personal biochemistry and reaching a fat-burning state. While ideal for all metabolic types, whey protein is particularly beneficial for muscle burners who can benefit from whey's ability to blunt the hormonal stress response and help the body gain, rather than burn, valuable muscle tissue.

Visit a health food or supplement store and the shelves will be packed with hundreds of different brands of whey protein powder, all claiming to be *the* miracle version. Read the labels and look for a whey-based protein powder that supplies at least 20g of whey protein in each scoop and is low in synthetic chemicals and fat-storing foods. (Avoid those with hydrogenated oils, high-fructose corn syrup, acesulfame, aspartame, and sucralose.) For those unfamiliar with whey protein, some good brands include our ME brand called The Meal and Jay Robb brand. The key with whey protein is to find one you like. We all have different tastes, so experiment until you find the brand and flavor you want.

Since it's inevitable that you'll consume some processed food, we came up with a simple formula that allows you to determine the hormonal impact of a food based on a ratio of carbohydrate/sugar to fiber and protein (fat being more neutral). Most people simply look at the number of calories on a food label, but that doesn't give you any information about hormonal impact. We start with carbohydrates rather than calories.

Carbohydrates can be divided into two categories—sugar and fiber. Anything that is not fiber is sugar and will create an insulin response, which is why the sugar designation on a nutrition label is pointless. Subtract the number of fiber grams from the total number of carbohydrate grams to give you the number of net carbs, or the carbs that will cause an insulin release. Then subtract the number of protein grams from the the net carb number. We call this number the hormonal carbs number because it's a direct reflection of the insulin to glucagon ratio, a prime determinant of fat burning. The number you get after subtracting the fiber and protein from the total carbohydrate should be less than or equal to 5, 10, or 15, depending on your burner type. The lower the number, the better for all types, and negative numbers are the best. Also, the number of fat grams on the label should be less than 15 and the sodium less than 200mg.

When buying whey protein powder, protein bars, and other packaged foods, use the diagram on page 119. After using this formula just a few times, you'll know how to read the labels and what to look for when you shop for food.

READING **FOOD LABELS**
THE *ME*™ WAY

1

HORMONAL CARBOHYDRATES

Sugar Burner ≤ **5**

Mixed Burner ≤ **10**

Muscle Burner ≤ **15**

2

TOTAL
FAT

≤ 15

Nutrition Facts

Serving Size 1/2 cup (114g)
Servings Per Container 4

Amount Per Serving

Calories 90   Calories from Fat 30

% **Daily Value***

Total Fat 3g	**5%**
Cholesterol 0g	**5%**
Sodium 3mg	**15%**
Total Carbohydrate 3g	**5%**
Dietary Fiber 3g	**12%**
Sugars 3g	
Protein 3g	

3

TOTAL
SODIUM

≤ **200**

METABOLIC
EFFECT

---

1 To find **hormonal carbohydrates**, find the total carbohydrate grams. Subtract the fiber grams (including any sugar alcohols). Finally, subtract the protein grams. You should be left with a number less than or between 5 to 15 depending on your type. The lower the number, the better Negative numbers are best.

2 **Total fat** content should be less than or equal to 15. Lower numbers are best. Avoid any foods with hydrogenated oils /trans-fats or mostly saturated fat. The higher the hormonal carbohydrate content of a food, the lower the fat should be and vice versa. Look for foods with higher amounts of mono *unsaturated* fats and omega-3 oils.

3 The amount of **sodium** in a food is an important component involved in fat loss. The sodium content of a packaged food should be less than or equal to 200mg. Look for foods with high potassium numbers and low sodium numbers. Try not to add extra salt to your foods.

FIBER

Fiber, one of the most useful tools in achieving a fat-burning physiology, is a blood sugar regulator, easing the flow of sugar into the body in a slow, controlled fashion, avoiding large surges in blood sugar, cravings, and hunger. This allows the body to secrete less insulin and therefore decreases fat storage.

Unfortunately, fiber is misunderstood by almost everyone, including doctors and other health professionals. If you want to know the fat-burning or fat-storing potential of a food, the ratio of sugar/starch to fiber is very important. The more sugar you have and the less fiber you have, the more insulin and fat storage that food will create. The less sugar/starch and the more fiber, the more of a fat-burning effect you will create. This is the reason vegetables and fruit are much better sources of fiber than grains (wheat, rice, etc.). Most people perceive grain as being the richest source of fiber, especially if it is whole grain. However, when you factor in the amount of sugar compared to fiber, it looks far less desirable. White bread has a very large amount of sugar and very little fiber and is a very poor choice for fat burning. Whole grains have less sugar and more fiber than white bread and therefore are the preferred choice.

However, most fruits have even less sugar and more fiber, and vegetables have an almost even amount of fiber compared to sugar. This means that in general vegetables and fruit will not only make you feel less hungry, but will create a hormonal effect that leads to fat burning, not storage.

- Eat 3 servings of vegetables and low-sugar fruit at each meal or 1 tablespoon of ME Fiber Complex with breakfast, lunch, or dinner.

Fiber:Sugar Ratio

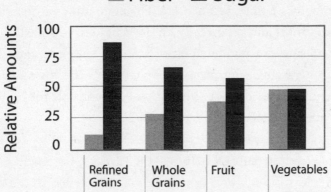

PHYTONUTRIENTS

The most exciting nutritional research is being done in the area of phytonutrients, the naturally occurring compounds found in plants. (The prefix "phyto" means *plant*.) Many of these compounds have profound effects on the body's physiology. While they are found in all vegetables and fruits, they also occur in wine, coffee, chocolate, spices, and other foods. What's even more exciting is that these compounds can be harnessed to unlock your fat-burning potential and keep you from regaining fat once it is lost.

The best way to take advantage of these compounds is to find rich sources that do not come in processed forms with loads of refined sugar. While fruit juices may contain some of these compounds, the amount of sugar in juices makes them less appropriate for fat loss. Eat foods that are as close to their original form as possible. Munch on apples instead of drinking sugar-laden apple juice. A handful of unsalted, roasted nuts and a square of dark chocolate are better for you than a candy bar. A healthy diet does not always equal a fat-loss diet. A fat-loss diet, however, is almost always a healthy diet.

Some of the best ways to get these valuable fat-burning compounds into the body is through berries. Blueberries, strawberries, raspberries, blackberries, and cherries contain large amounts of these compounds and aid the body's ability to burn fat. The compounds in berries are called anthocyanins and act directly on the genes responsible for determining whether or not you burn fat or store it. They accomplish this by directly interacting with genes present in fat cells, turning on an important enzyme called AMP kinase that is responsible for switching the body from sugar burning to fat burning.

GREEN AND BLACK TEA

Another phytonutrient compound is found in green and black teas. These teas come from the actual tea plant (*Camillia senensis*). (Don't confuse these with herbal teas, which may contain some green or black tea, but are usually made from herbs, flowers, and other plants.) Epigallocatechin gallate or EGCG, a compound found in tea plants, has a fat-burning effect in the body. Green tea is able to interact with your metabolism at the level of the liver and fat cells. As with the berry compounds, this effect stems from the compounds in green tea being able to speak directly to the genes responsible for producing fat-burning enzymes. While green tea has the highest concentration of these phytonutrient compounds, oolong tea and other black tea varieties also deliver favorable effects. When it comes to caffeine, black teas have the most, followed by green.

HERBAL TEAS

Herbal teas made from herbs, spices, and flowers—any plant other than the actual tea plant—also contain phytonutrients. Many of them, such as chamomile, lemon balm, and Siberian ginseng teas, reduce stress and calm the mind. The compounds present in these teas also relax the nervous system, acting in a similar fashion to some prescription anti-anxiety or antidepressant medications. When buying herbal teas, read the labels carefully and choose those that are pure herbs and not combined with green or black teas. Hot or cold, enjoy 3 to 6 cups of pure herbal tea a day whether you're a sugar, mixed, or muscle burner.

CONDIMENTS AND SPICES

Most people think of condiments and spices as food flavor boosters, having little, if anything, to do with fat burning. It turns out that these ingredients do play important roles in metabolism. When you eat a salad with a vinegar-based dressing, a signal is sent to your brain indicating that you are full, which drastically curtails the amount of food you consume at one time. Vinegar also synergistically decreases the insulin released from a meal rich in carbohydrates. Studies show that vinegar can decrease the insulin response of a meal by more than 20 percent and increase insulin sensitivity by 34 percent. Since insulin is a primary fat-storing hormone, this effect means less fat storage. Vinegar helps you feel full more quickly and prolongs the amount of time you feel full. This can significantly reduce cravings and the need to overeat, while at the same time lowering fat-storing hormones and allowing you to burn fat for a longer period of time.

Readily available cinnamon, chiles, and fresh ginger directly impact the body's fat-burning ability. For centuries, Traditional Chinese Medicine doctors promoted these warming ingredients as fat-burning aids, and scientific research confirms those recommendations. From a metabolic point of view, these ingredients act as metabolic messengers and have the ability to affect hunger, lower fat-storing hormones, and make fat more likely to be burned rather than stored.

○　○　○

Spice It Up

Cinnamon, cayenne, and chiles are great metabolic messengers, but they are only good if they are fresh and used on a regular basis. If the spices in your cabinet are more than 6 months old, toss them out and buy fresh ones. Keep them in a cool, dark place—not on a spice rack above the stove or exposed to sunlight. Use them regularly; a dash of cinnamon in your hot cocoa once a year won't be of any help.

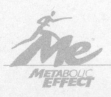

CHOCOLATE AND COCOA

Yup, that's right. Chocolate is a fat-burning food. But keep in mind that this may not be the type of chocolate you are thinking of; 100 percent cocoa powder, unsweetened and loaded with phytonutrients, can aid you in fat-loss efforts. The major benefit of cocoa (the main ingredient in chocolate) is in its ability to directly affect the pleasure centers in the brain. The compound phenylethylamine (PEA) helps you feel satisfied, motivated, and energized. This effect cannot be overstated. The most well-intentioned and well-planned goals often fail due to neglect of the motivational aspects of the process. The compounds in cocoa are an amazing asset for all types and greatly enhance the metabolic effect. See the recipe for the cocoa drink on page 186, used by cultures for centuries to aid health and control fat gain. Drink it with pleasure and without guilt.

All chocolate bars are made with sugar and will raise insulin levels, so it is preferable that you not eat commercial chocolate bars. Muscle burners and mixed burners, however, can eat two small squares of dark chocolate (not milk or white). Remember, two small squares, not a candy bar or a scoop of chocolate ice cream. Sorry, sugar burners, but you need to avoid that extra sugar, and given your metabolic makeup, you're rarely able to eat just two. Stick with the cocoa drink for best results.

WATER

Some people advocate drinking as much water as you can throughout the day, while others say you get all you need from food and other beverages. As with most things, the truth lies somewhere in the middle.

When we talk about achieving the Metabolic Effect, the ultimate goal is to reach a state of optimal health. In most cases, although you won't become clinically dehydrated by drinking beverages other than water, it's difficult to reach your fat-loss goals without plenty of this super nutrient. Water is one of your greatest allies in achieving the Metabolic Effect.

Drinking water is also a valuable tool for controlling hunger. A study in the *Journal of the American Dietetics Association* (July 2008) showed that participants who drank large glasses of water immediately before meals were able to significantly blunt their hunger and eat less. Another study in the journal *Obesity* (November 2008) showed that increased water intake in obese women was associated with lower weight, independent of diet or exercise.

It's important to drink water and remain hydrated to stay healthy. Until the last several generations, people remained hydrated because their sodium intake was low and their potassium intake was higher, negating the need to drink water constantly. People didn't carry around containers with water until bottled water became a profit center for beverage companies and Americans increased their sodium intake by eating processed foods.

Water means water. Not a fluorescent-colored sports drink loaded with brominates, vegetable oil, and high-fructose corn syrup. Not artificially flavored and sweetened bottled water. We mean plain water either from the tap, if your local water supply is clean, or filtered through a pitcher or sink attachment. Water filters are becoming more of a necessity since tap water frequently contains traces of chemicals, drugs, and hormones that can have an effect on your health and your metabolism. Many of these compounds can impact the ability to burn fat.

It's not a simple matter of water in, water out, as some experts believe; there's a dynamic, complex process going on that involves the types of fats present in cell membranes, the relative amounts of minerals in the diet, and even the size of the water clusters that are consumed. As with everything else, how much water you should drink depends on your individual makeup. Too little water results in dehydration, sodium retention, and slowed fat burning. Too much water depletes the body of electrolytes, which also can lead to dehydration and slowed fat burning.

Listen to your body and drink the right amount of water for you. To guarantee adequate hydration, use the following guidelines:

- Coffee, alcohol, fruit juice, and sodas do not count as water. For every 8 ounces of these liquids you consume, drink an equivalent amount of water.
- Filtered water is a necessity due to all the chemicals (chlorine, fluorine) and other substances found in our water supply that can take their toll on liver metabolism. We mean filtered, not bottled, water unless your tap water is undrinkable even after it has been filtered. Purchase a water-filtration pitcher or faucet to save money and turn tap water into a clean refreshment.
- Drink enough water so that your urine is consistently light yellow or almost clear in color.

SWEETENERS

You've already learned how detrimental processed and refined sugars are when it comes to fat burning, but everyone occasionally needs to satisfy that sweet tooth. There are a number of naturally occurring sweeteners that you can use without worry.

We don't recommend artificial or synthetic sweeteners such as NutraSweet, Equal, etc., since their long-term effects on humans are unknown. Studies show that these sugar substitutes can increase your hunger between meals and that even the taste of them can cause the release of fat-storing hormones in the body.

Not to worry, the best sweeteners are ones that have been a natural part of the human diet for centuries.

Agave nectar or *syrup* comes from the same cactus plant used in making tequila. This sweetener has become quite popular since it's considered "natural," but its molecular structure is exactly the same as that of the high-fructose corn syrup used in sodas and other foods. It should not be used as a sweetener.

Erythritol (pronounced e-*rith*-ra-tall) is a sugar alcohol—it tastes like sugar, but has almost no calories. It is naturally occurring in fruit and does not create a fat-storing hormone response. Erythritol also acts as a prebiotic, a compound that feeds the healthy bacteria living in our digestive tract, and can aid in digestion. Brand names are ZSweet, Zero, and Sweet Simplicity. Two teaspoons of erythritol powder equals the sweetness of 1 tablespoon of sugar.

Honey, a favorite sweetener of health food proponents, is a healthier alternative to refined sugars, but it acts like sugar by increasing insulin production, raising blood sugar levels, and switching the body back into sugar-burning mode. While muscle burners can use 1 teaspoon of honey once or twice each day, more than that will disrupt fat burning.

Xylitol (zi-lit-tol) is a natural compound occurring in the human body. Humans actually make several grams of this compound daily. Commercially made from inherently sweet birch tree bark or corncobs, xylitol powder looks and tastes like sugar. Xylitol has a minimal effect on fat-storing hormones and may actually aid the body's ability to make muscle and bone. It even helps protect against tooth decay and upper respiratory tract infections. Like vinegar, xylitol slows gastric emptying, which results in staying satisfied for longer after a meal. The trade names are ME LeanSweet XyloSweet, and the Ultimate Sweetener, and you'll find them in the nutritional supplement area of health food stores. Use a ratio of one to one in place of sugar.

Stevia, also known as sweet leaf, is a plant native to South America. Consumed by humans for thousands of years, stevia is 300 times sweeter than sugar. Stevia has no calories and does not affect fat-storing hormone production. In addition, it may have antiviral effects. It is available as an extract that comes with a dropper or as a powder; the extract may need to be diluted even further. A little bit of stevia goes a long way, so start with a small amount. Brand names include SweetLeaf, Truvia, and PureVia.

WHAT TO EAT FOR YOUR BURNER TYPE

We could focus this entire book on eating foods with metabolically active compounds, but the important thing to understand is that every single time you eat, you make the choice to increase or decrease the fat-burning effects of foods. Some of these food messengers are better for different metabolic types, as we explain below. By integrating these metabolic food factors into meals and snacks, you can boost the fat-burning effects of your diet.

Sugar Burners

If you're a sugar burner, you want to eat foods that keep your liver and pancreas healthy, warm up your body, and keep you satisfied between meals.

HUNGER
Vinegar and Fiber

If you're a sugar burner, you love food and you love to eat, yet you have an exaggerated fat-storing hormone response to your meals. To compensate, include vinegar in your diet. Vinegar slows down the time it takes for food to leave the stomach and decreases the insulin-releasing effects of a meal, which means that you will become fuller faster, stay full longer, and increase your fat-burning mechanism. To take advantage of vinegar's positive effects, make your own dressing with plenty of vinegar and less oil than in a traditional vinaigrette (see page 197 for recipe), and eat your salad before the rest of your meal.

- Make salad dressings with vinegar rather than lemon juice. Choose from red wine, balsamic, herb-flavored, or fruit-flavored vinegars. Whisk together 1 teaspoon or more of vinegar and 1 tablespoon of olive oil for a large individual

salad. The more vinegar used, the better the response.
- Italians have known the health benefits of vinegar for centuries; they often drink a shot of their best-quality balsamic vinegar before meals. Use top-notch balsamic vinegar (made only from grapes and aged for at least twelve years). Enjoy a shot or add a few drops to a glass of sparkling water.

ENERGY
Cocoa and Coffee

Drinking coffee imparts short-term bursts of energy, often followed by energy lows, cravings, and increased hunger. Drinking coffee in the morning frequently results in increased cravings and eating in the evening. Cocoa, on the other hand, provides sustained energy, decreases hunger, and enhances motivation, with fewer food cravings. See page 186 for a cocoa drink.

- Treat yourself to 1 cup of black coffee before your morning workout.
- 1 to 3 cups of cocoa each day provide energy.

CRAVINGS
Cocoa, Fiber, and Xylitol

If you're a sugar burner, you know you love to eat. Sugar burners often crave sweets, but will eat just about anything when they are hungry. Cocoa, fiber-rich fruits and vegetables, fiber supplements, and xylitol used as a sweetener reduce those cravings.

- Cocoa drinks decrease those sweet cravings by stimulating the pleasure centers in the brain. Satisfy those cravings with cocoa drinks.
- Eating fiber, by which we mean vegetables and low-sugar

fruits, causes the release of specific hormones that tell the brain when we are full and when to stop eating. Fiber also slows down gastric transit and increases gastric distention, which means that food passes out of the stomach at a slower pace, causing a decrease in a hormonal response such as producing insulin. Until recent times, human beings ate as much as 100g of fiber per day. Today the average American barely eats 20 to 30g.

It's best to get all nutrients from natural food sources, which is why we recommend eating at least 5 servings of fiber-rich vegetables and fruit every day. Unfortunately, most people just can't seem to get 5 servings of fiber into their daily meals. If you're one of those people, then we suggest taking a fiber supplement such as ME Fiber Complex™ in powder form. ME Fiber Complex™ is a combination of fibers derived from fruits, vegetables, roots, seeds, and tree extracts. ME Fiber Complex™ was created with the features of a Paleolithic diet in mind, which is what our human physiology is adapted from. Dissolve 1 tablespoon ME Fiber Complex™ in an 8-ounce glass of water before drinking. Whenever increasing fiber content in your diet, do so slowly so the body can adapt. Start with ½ teaspoon per day, increasing the amount by ½ teaspoon every 4 to 5 days until the daily dose is 1 to 3 tablespoons.

- Xylitol provides a touch of sweetness while promoting a feeling of fullness.

FAT BURNING
Green Tea, Omega-3 Oils, and Warm Spices

Sugar burners need all the help they can get to reach a fat-burning state and stay there.

- Green tea works to aid fat loss, and much of its effect is seen in the liver, a prime area of dysfunction for sugar burners, which is often compromised in its ability to regulate fat burning.

- Omega-3 oils coax the body to burn fat at the level of the genes, giving a much-needed boost to the sluggish sugar burner's metabolism. Eat fish and other rich sources of omega-3 oils. Use flaxseed meal on salads and oatmeal, or take a fish oil supplement every day.
- Warm spices—cinnamon, chiles, cayenne, and ginger—also speed the metabolic processes of a sugar burner, stimulating improved digestion, the assimilation of food, and enhanced fat burning.

Mixed Burners

Unlike sugar burners or muscle burners, you have no specific metabolic tendencies, but instead are pushed more toward sugar or muscle burning based on your lifestyle. All the food messengers will be beneficial for you, but some will aid you more than others.

HUNGER
Fiber and Whey Protein Powder

Keeping your body from being hungry is really a matter of making sure you are getting adequate fiber and protein. Both whey protein and fruit and vegetable fibers have the unique benefits of simultaneously affecting hunger hormones and controlling the ratio of fat-storing versus fat-burning hormones.

- Drink your protein shakes.
- Try to eat three vegetables and/or low-sugar fruits with each meal, always eating more vegetables than fruit. See the mixed burner food list on page 64.

ENERGY
Green and Black Tea

Green and black teas have small amounts of stimulating caffeine along with other food messengers such as theanine that have a relaxing and calming affect on the mixed burner's mind. Together, caffeine and theanine create a relaxed but energized state that is ideal for staying focused, motivated, and balanced.

• Drink 1 to 6 cups of green or black tea per day.

CRAVINGS
Cocoa

As a mixed burner, you probably bounce back and forth between craving salt and craving sugar, depending on your stress levels and other factors. Reaching for a cocoa drink instead of cookies or potato chips will balance your biochemistry and prevent those salty and/or sweet cravings.

• Keep a container of raw organic cocoa powder on hand and make the cocoa drink on page 186 when food cravings set in.
• As a mixed burner, you can eat two small squares of dark chocolate (not milk or white) with 70 percent cocoa once or twice a day. Lucky you!

FAT BURNING
Green Tea, Omega-3 Oils, and Cocoa

Green tea works in two ways for mixed burners. First, as you have learned, it turns on fat burning at the level of the genes. Second, green tea has a compound called theanine, an amino acid that helps reduce the body's reaction to stress. Since mixed burners can be pulled in either the sugar burner or muscle burner direction depending on foods and stress, green tea is a powerful ally that works on both fronts.

Omega-3 oils burn fat at the level of the genes and can be of benefit for mixed burners. Fish, a rich source of omega-3 oils, is a great choice. While flaxseed oil does not pack as powerful an omega-3 punch as fish, it does provide some benefit. Flax meal has minuscule amounts of omega-3 oil, but it is a significant source of fiber. Take a fish oil supplement daily.

Cocoa has unique actions that stabilize blood sugar, blunt cravings, and boost energy, all of which help the mixed burner stay in balance.

Muscle Burners

Muscle burners are unique in that their metabolism is hyperresponsive to stress and often prefers to run off the energy derived from the central nervous system, which means they can often oversecrete the stress hormones cortisol, adrenaline, and noradrenaline. While this keeps them thin, it also means they are using up valuable muscle. The following food messengers most beneficial to muscle burners are geared toward making the nervous system more efficient and less reactive, while allowing the adrenal glands to produce a steadier flow of energy.

ENERGY
Herbal Teas

It's not unusual to find muscle burners who live on coffee and cigarettes or alcohol. Many like the up-and-down buzz they get from these stimulants and depressants. Muscle burners are characterized by an exaggerated stress response and are usually what we call dopamine dominant. Dopamine is a neurohormone released by the brain that helps us feel focused, motivated, and energized. It's also a pleasure-seeking hormone that contributes to addictive behavior such as stimulant and illegal drug use. The use of chamomile, lemon balm, and Siberian ginseng teas go a long way toward balancing out the wired but tired feeling that muscle burners often have.

- Drink herbal teas throughout the day, with more ginseng
  in the morning and more chamomile and lemon balm in the
  afternoon and evening. Muscle burners benefit from skullcap,
  lavender, and passionflower teas. Bedtime by Yogi Teas is one
  of our favorites for muscle burners.

HUNGER
Whey Protein Powder

Muscle burners often go for long periods of time without eating, but once hunger sets in, they become ravenous, indiscriminate, and eat everything in sight. Whey protein powder not only fights hunger, it also lowers the stress hormones cortisol, adrenaline, and noradrenaline. At the same time, it raises serotonin levels, which tend to settle the sometimes overactive minds of muscle burners. And the one thing muscle burners require more than anything else is a steady supply of amino acids to keep them from losing muscle and developing a thin, flabby look.

- Keep a can of flavored—chocolate, vanilla, strawberry,
  fruit—whey protein powder on hand and stir a scoop or
  two into an 8-ounce glass of water. A glass of water with
  whey protein powder is a good snack to keep muscle burners
  from using up their muscle tissue and controls those binges
  that tend to occur later in the day. Many of our clients keep
  shaker bottles in their cars or at their desks so they can shake
  up a quick protein drink when cravings hit.

CRAVINGS
Cocoa and Whey Protein

Cocoa is king when it comes to blunting food cravings. Cocoa is rich in magnesium, a mineral frequently used up in muscle burners due to their overreactive stress response. Again, whey protein fights cravings in muscle burners due to its ability to supply the body with the essential amino acids that are the building blocks for muscle and brain hormones like dopamine, serotonin, and others. Cravings in muscle burners can often be traced back to a lack of a specific amino acid (tyrosine, tryptophan, leucine, or glutamine), which are necessary for producing brain chemicals. Whey protein supplies these amino acids along with a whole host of others.

- Enjoy 1 to 3 cups of cocoa every day.
- Make sure you get 50g to 100g of protein per day.
  Supplement your protein intake with 2 to 4 protein shakes throughout the day.

FAT BURNING
Green Tea

Green tea is a useful fat-burning aid because stress hormones can often affect the liver's ability to balance blood sugar and burn fat. Green tea works at the level of the liver to help the body more efficiently regulate its fuel and burn fat more readily.

- Drink 1 to 5 cups of green tea every day.

○ ○ ○

Functional Foods

People often wait too long between meals and then are too hungry to prepare foods for a healthy meal. A functional food is one that provides health benefits beyond its nutritional value. Functional foods provide a key benefit by ensuring that there are always healthy eating options available. Vegetable and fruit powdered concentrates, protein bars and shakes, and fiber supplements are some of the basic functional foods followers of the fat-loss lifestyle will need. These foods effectively mimic the nutritional components of the historic hunter-gatherer diet. Vegetables and fruit concentrates, cocoa powder, protein shakes, and fiber supplements travel easily and can be quickly mixed with water in a shaker bottle. Keep protein bars in your tote bag, briefcase, or car, and at work. The smart use of convenient functional foods like these ensures that you always have easy access to healthy foods that serve your metabolism and keep you in the fat-burning zone.

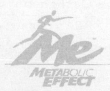

CHAPTER SIX

THE TRANSFORMATION WORKOUT

The first part of your workout in the Metabolic Transformation section is similar to the one you did throughout the Metabolic Spark Stage, except that you will do only 8 back-to-back reps from the 4 hybrid exercises (page 85). Rest as necessary and resume the workout for 20 minutes as soon as you are ready, picking up where you left off. You will also be using heavier weights with fewer repetitions and adding supersets to boost the amount of HGH and testosterone released during your workout. Together these are two of the most effective strategies for building muscle and burning fat we have ever seen.

The Transformation Workout looks like this:

- Warm up for 1 to 2½ minutes and cool down for 2½ to 4 minutes (see page 75).
- Increase the amount of weight lifted.
- Decrease the number of reps from 12 to 8.
- Do the hybrid circuit for 20 minutes.
- Add 5 minutes of supersets.
- Perform the Transformation Workout 3 times per week.

INCREASE THE AMOUNT OF WEIGHT LIFTED

The amount of weight lifted is different for everyone, so we've come up with an easy formula to help you figure out how much you should lift in the Metabolic Transformation Workout. Choose a weight that allows you to do just 3 perfect bicep curls and then cut that weight in half as you did in the Spark Stage. Then add 5 to 10 pounds in each dumbbell.

Your workout performance determines whether the amount of weight being used should be increased, decreased, or remain the same. Once you choose an initial amount of weight, your goal is to complete 4 to 5 rounds of the hybrid exercise circuit in 20 minutes. If you're able to complete 5 or more rounds, then increase the amount of weight at your next workout. If you're unable to complete at least 4 rounds, then decrease the amount of weight at your next workout. Increase or decrease the weight by 2½ to 5 pounds for each dumbbell.

Using more weight means you have to pay special attention to your form when doing the exercises; the additional weight will also force you to rest more often.

The ME™ *Transformation* Workout is
designed to increase the Metabolic Burn, increase HGH and testosterone to aid the gain of muscle.

PART 1

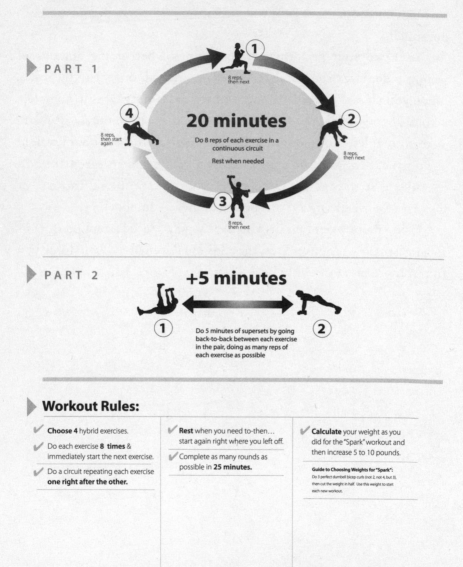

20 minutes

Do 8 reps of each exercise in a continuous circuit

Rest when needed

1 — 8 reps, then next

2 — 8 reps, then next

3 — 8 reps, then next

4 — 8 reps, then start again

PART 2

+5 minutes

1   Do 5 minutes of supersets by going back-to-back between each exercise in the pair, doing as many reps of each exercise as possible   2

Workout Rules:

✔ **Choose 4** hybrid exercises.

✔ Do each exercise **8 times** & immediately start the next exercise.

✔ Do a circuit repeating each exercise **one right after the other.**

✔ **Rest** when you need to-then... start again right where you left off.

✔ Complete as many rounds as possible in **25 minutes.**

✔ **Calculate** your weight as you did for the "Spark" workout and then increase 5 to 10 pounds.

Guide to Choosing Weights for "Spark":
Do 3 perfect dumbell bicep curls (not 2, not 4, but 3), then cut the weight in half. Use this weight to start each new workout.

ADD SUPERSETS

The last 5 minutes of the Transformation Workout includes the addition of supersets, an advanced exercise technique designed to generate a "burn" in the muscles, a feeling that you can't continue doing the exercise any longer.

Supersets are super simple. They consist of 2 exercises done back-to-back with little or no rest to bring the muscle to full fatigue. The superset technique increases fat burning and muscle building by putting increased demand on the muscles and harnessing the direct power of muscle molecules.

In the superset section you will choose 1 pair of exercises from 4 categories:

- Chest and Back

or

- Legs

or

- Biceps and Triceps

or

- Core and Shoulders

For your supersets, you will first decrease the weight you are using by ½ of the total weight. If you're using two 15-pound dumbbells for the hybrid exercises, then use two 7½-pound weights for the supersets. If you selected an exercise that uses only your own body weight (like a push-up), drop to your knees if toe push-ups are too hard. Do each exercise in your chosen pair for as many repetitions as you can until you simply can't perform another one. Complete one exercise immediately followed by the other in back-to-back succession for as many rounds as possible in 5 minutes. As with the hybrid section of the workout, push until you can't do any more and rest until you can continue. Your goal in doing the supersets is to go to failure in each exercise as many times as possible and take only enough rest to allow you to continue. By the end of 5 minutes you may be able to do only a few reps of each exercise before stopping and moving on to the other exercise. This is perfect and right where you should be!

Unlike the hybrid exercises, superset exercises isolate specific areas of the body. Many people choose superset pairs that address their trouble spots, such as crunches for the midsection and squats for the legs and buttocks. Just make sure you choose a different superset for each workout so that all 4 pairs are done every 4 workouts.

Reset your watch or timer for this 5-minute superset.

Remember, supersets are 2 exercises done back-to-back without rest. Choose 1 pair (2 exercises) of the following superset exercises. For example, if you want to focus on your core and shoulders, choose the crunches and shoulder press pairing. Alternate back and forth between those two for 5 minutes. Be sure to choose the supersets in sequence so that each one is done every 4 workouts. Here are the supersets:

Pairing 1: Push-ups and Rows

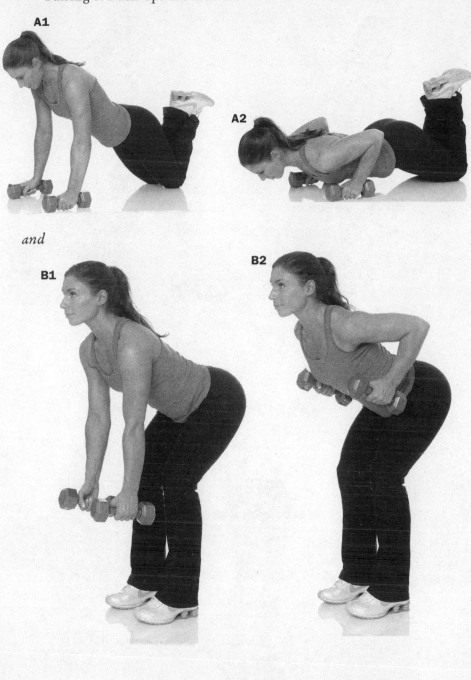

and

Pairing 2: Lungs and Squats

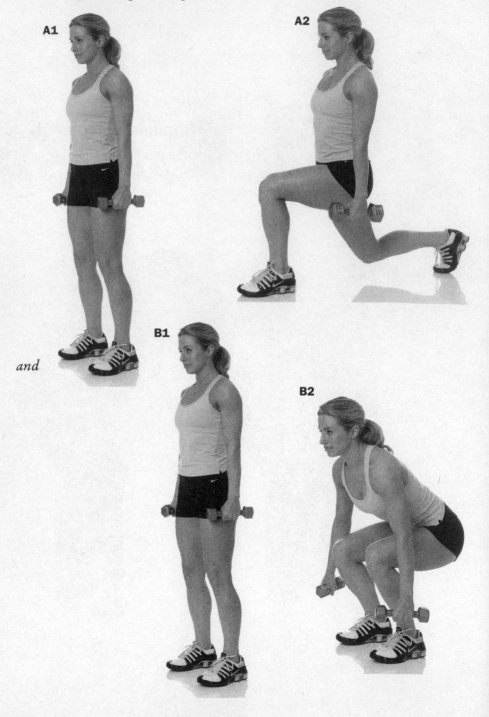

and

Pairing 3: Bicep Curls and Tricep Dips

A1

A2

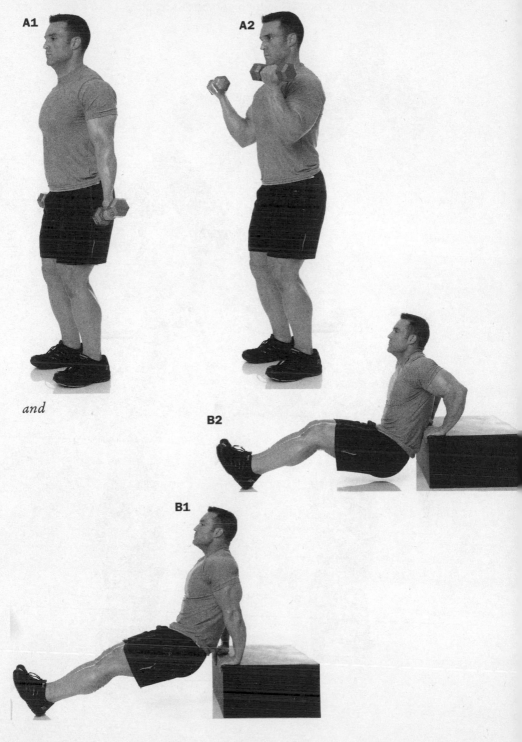

and

B2

B1

Pairing 4: Chest Press/Crunch and Shoulder Presses

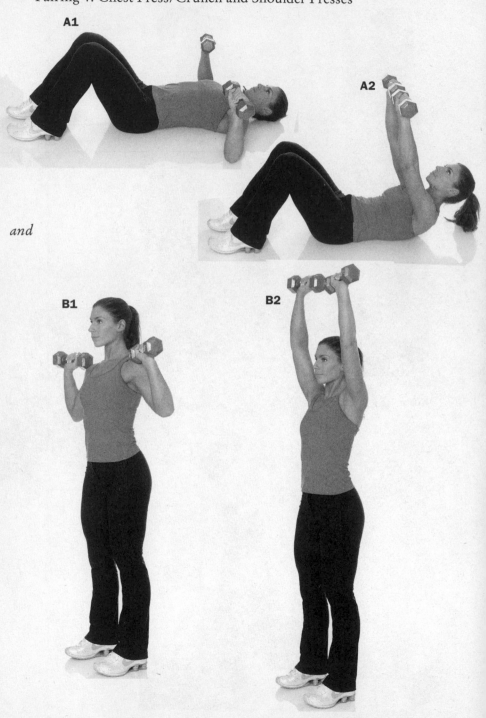

A1

A2

and

B1

B2

SAMPLE TRANSFORMATION SEGMENT

Let's say you choose chest press/crunches and shoulder presses for your first 5-minute superset segment. Here's how it will go:

- Do chest press/crunches until you can't do one more. When doing crunches, focus on contracting your abdominal muscles.
- Get up immediately. Using the same weights, do shoulder presses until you can't do any more.
- Holding the weights, lie down on the floor, and do chest press/crunches until you can't continue.
- Get back up immediately, pick up the weights, and do shoulder presses until you reach a 4 on the exertion scale.
- Continue this sequence, going back and forth between chest press/crunches and shoulder presses for 5 minutes. When the 5 minutes are up, stop wherever you are in the sequence. Your segment is finished.

If this seems confusing, write down the sequences on index cards to take to the gym until the routine becomes natural. And it will once you do them a couple of times.

For those who are more advanced, feel free to adjust some of the superset exercises by adding weight or doing more difficult exercises like one-leg squats, half squats, or squat jumps in place of regular squats.

30-Minute Transformation Workout Sample

Here's what your Transformation Workout might look like:

Choose four exercises selected from hybrid exercises (pages 85–103) such as:

Chest Press/Crunch
Lunge/Side Raise
Squat/Row
Lunge/Curl/Press

Repeat continuously, doing 8 reps of each exercise back-to-back for 20 minutes.

Choose one exercise pair from the Transformation Supersets (pages 143–146), such as chest press/crunch and shoulder presses:

Chest Press/Crunch: until complete failure, then
Shoulder Press: until complete failure

Repeat these 2 exercises, doing each one back-to-back to failure continuously for 5 minutes.

The 20-Minute Transformation Workout Reminder

· 1- to 2-minute warm-up
· 20-minute section of hybrid exercises, increased amount of weight, and lowering the number of repetitions from 12 to 8
· 5-minute superset exercise session
· Do this workout 3 times per week.

HOW YOU KNOW THE METABOLIC TRANSFORMATION IS WORKING

During the Metabolic Transformation you'll see major changes in your body. The continuous process involves the mastery of the dietary and exercise practices of both the Spark Stage and the Transformation Stage. As you progress through the Transformation during the coming days, weeks, and months, you will see the powerful effect and results that your hormones have when it comes to burning fat and building muscle. We find that successfully mastering the Transformation Stage depends on how committed you are to the ME program. You've already seen the dramatic results from the Spark Stage in just a few short months. The Transformation Stage will take another 2 to 3 months while your body completes the remodeling of your muscle mass metabolic machinery.

You'll see dramatic changes in your physique. Your clothes will be too big. Your arms, legs, and other areas will have a sculpted, toned look. Your skin will be plump, but not fleshy. Your eyes will be bright and clear. You'll reach a happy state of awareness about your body that you never had before. You'll have increased stamina and plenty of energy. You'll sleep deeply and throughout the night. You'll be less moody and less reliant on stimulants like coffee and depressants like alcohol. You'll make wise choices when it comes to food so you continue to burn fat and build muscle. You'll automatically know what to eat and what not to eat to drive your internal metabolic mechanisms. You'll be motivated to continue your workouts. You'll feel more athletic and look forward to hiking, biking, swimming, and other physical activities with friends and family. You'll have an intimate understanding that becoming and staying lean, healthy, and fit is about making choices that directly impact your hormonal biochemistry.

You have achieved the Metabolic Effect, that optimal state of hormonal balance that sustains energy, health, and well-being.

Weight Training: The Fountain of Youth

In 1513 Spanish explorer Ponce de Leon landed in Florida in search of the fountain of youth. While he never found it, humans remain obsessed with living a youthful, vigorous life. Injections, hair replacement, raw food and vegan diets, body augmentation, "guaranteed" nutritional supplements, and exotic rain forest herbs are today's equivalents of de Leon's sixteenth-century mission. These zealous pursuits are doomed to fail as people achieve only short-lived gains while the body continues to age, sag, and degenerate, resulting in a weak skeleton, forgetful mind, and a body devoid of muscle, strength, and vitality.

This isn't a very pleasant picture, but it doesn't have to be this way. On a trip to Los Angeles, California, we were in a gym and saw something that flew in the face of common knowledge related to aging. We instantly recognized a once-famous bodybuilder. We knew he had to be at least 70 years old, but to look at his face he could easily pass for 50 or even 40. And his body was unbelievable. He was no longer the heavily muscled bodybuilder of his younger days, but he still had more muscle than 99 percent of 20-year-olds walking on the street today. He was not bent over, slow moving, or cautious in his actions. He was upright, strong, and agile, stepping over dumbbells and doing barbell squats with ease and agility. At first, we thought it had to be his son or a look-alike, but it wasn't. And we found out that he was actually 77.

This got us thinking. If he had defied the laws of aging, surely there had to be others who had been in the weight-lifting game for so long and continued to look and function on a different plane from the rest of us. On the other hand, it's difficult to find the same results in other sports. Every now and then you may read about a distance runner who is still active in his seventies, yet as impressive as he is, he doesn't have the same youthful appearance as his weight-training counterparts do. What is it about weight training that produces these results?

In the world of nature, you are either in growth or decay. You can't be in both states at once; it just doesn't work that way. Decay is the very definition of aging. The body parts break down, joints give out, skin loses its natural moisture and elasticity, bones become brittle, and muscle dries and shrivels. Growth is the opposite. The joints become stronger, skin stays moist and firm, bones remain sturdy, muscles stay strong, and the nerves stay responsive.

It's well known in science that aging is associated with a sharp decline in circulating hormones and muscle mass. This occurrence has always been seen as the inevitable consequence of becoming old. But now research is showing that the body is much more resilient. It seems that lifestyle plays a bigger role than age when it comes to declining hormones and muscle function. Science is now proving resistance training to be the ultimate antiaging strategy. To understand how this works, it is necessary to understand what is happening to our muscles and hormones as we age.

The word "sarcopenia" refers to the loss of muscle, strength, and function, a process that begins in the third or fourth decade of life and accelerates dramatically after age 70.

For a muscle to function correctly, there is a closely orchestrated association between that muscle and the nerves that spark muscular activity, known as "innervation." In sarcopenia, the loss of functioning muscle is initiated by a loss of nerve innervation to what are known as fast-twitch muscle fibers (FT fibers). These muscle fibers are unique because they are larger, have faster firing rates, are quicker to contract, and produce more muscle force than slow-twitch muscle fibers (ST fibers). Sarcopenia is characterized by a replacement of FT fibers with ST fibers, resulting in less muscle mass and less efficient muscle function.

Looking closely at the mechanism and thinking about why FT fibers are lost as we age, the conclusion is a lack of high-intensity lifting. Weight lifting with purposeful muscular contractions is the only way to increase and maintain FT fibers. Endurance exercise—running, walking, swimming—does not affect FT fibers, yet it is the primary form of exercise advised by health professionals. Cardiovascular exercise like running and biking is an ST fiber–dominant activity and, therefore, can never replace the loss of the strength given by FT fibers. Look at endurance athletes at the top of their game. They may be lean and impressive, but their lack of muscle is striking. The gaunt appearance of these athletes is proof that muscle will not reappear with an aerobic exercise regimen.

It is obvious what is happening. Activity declines significantly for people as they age, and popular expert opinion has dictated a cardiovascular-centered exercise approach for decades. The combination of these two trends has been devastating to human muscle function and therefore has drastically affected aging. For centuries, humans had to lift, haul, push, and carry on a daily basis. Trading in our lifting-centered physical labor for running shoes was an ill-advised move.

When most people think of hormones, they think of the sex steroids like estrogen and progesterone, but hormonal action in the body does not stop at reproduction. In fact, all the hormones in the body impact aging and are affected directly or indirectly by weight training. The unique symphony of hormonal influence induced by weight training unleashes a powerful growth stimulus that far surpasses any imitation hormonal therapy. Hormones released from resistance training determine muscle growth, affect skin texture and tone, build bone, and repair damage. These hormones include growth hormone, IGF-1 (a potent hormone that affects muscle growth), and testosterone, among others.

It has been shown that older and aging individuals have much lower levels of these hormones when compared with their younger counter-parts. After about age 30, levels begin to fall, resulting in a significant loss of muscle mass along with degeneration of joints and other tissue. Science has long held that this is an inevitable consequence of aging. But is it? Are we destined to lose our hormonal growth potential and vitality, or is our sedentary lifestyle to blame?

Weight training, unlike other forms of exercise, will not only keep us from losing our valuable growth-producing hormones, but can actually replace them once they are gone. A study published online at the *Public Library of Science* (May 2007) shows the dramatic potential for resistance training to reverse the aging effect in muscle. Twenty-five seniors were compared with their younger counterparts in regard to muscle function and then engaged in a 6-month resistance-training program. The research-ers looked at more than five hundred genes related to muscle and aging. At the beginning of the study, the elderly subjects were shown to have dramatically weaker muscle and much lower gene activity. At the end of the study, researchers saw an enormous increase in muscle strength and a dramatic reversal of gene activity in the senior participants.

Seeing the effects of resistance training on preventing and reversing muscle loss and maintaining growth hormone production is compelling, but what about other changes encountered in aging? The loss of bone, skin tone, sexual potency, and brain function are also greatly impacted. Several studies have shown the potential of resistance training not only to maintain bone mass but increase it, something aerobic exercise has never been able to accomplish. In addition, when it comes to avoiding falls and maintaining balance and coordination, a serious concern for seniors, the strength and speed of fast-twitch fibers become mandatory. Resistance training is the only true means of building muscle and bone while at the same time developing functional parameters of balance and coordination to avoid falls.

A study in the *Journal of Experimental Gerontology* (September 2007) highlighted the profound impact decreased growth hormone and sex hormone levels have on the youthfulness of skin. In addition to skin texture and tone, weight training tightens the skin through the effect muscle has on the underlying connective tissue. This is the reason the skin of weight lifters is taut and feels firm to the touch. Women who opt for cardio over weights are missing the benefits of better skin texture and firmness.

Finally, two of our society's biggest fears are loss of memory and sexual function. Both brain function and sexual potency are greatly enhanced by weight training. Two 2007 studies, one from the Karolinska Institute and the other from Columbia University Medical Center, show how exercise regenerates brain cells and improves mood and memory. While this is not an effect unique to weight training, the added hormonal stimulus weight training provides has been shown to improve self-esteem over and above that provided by cardiovascular training. This holds true in sexual potency as well. Weight training benefits performance and desire in both males and females.

When it comes to antiaging, weight training is key and must replace the cardiovascular-centered approach of most exercise programs. To see how far we have taken the aerobics-in-place-of-weights paradigm, all you need to do is drive through a residential area shortly after work or peer into your local gym. What you will see on the streets is one runner after the next struggling along in a desperate attempt to halt the aging process. The story in the gym is no different, with the vast majority of exercisers occupying the cardio and aerobics room over the weight-training section. Like Ponce de Leon, the search for the fountain of youth proves futile for these exercisers. The real fountain of youth lies in the pursuit of weight training, which, when done correctly, is also aerobic in nature. Weights alone induce the hormonal- and muscle-changing effects that have the potential to remake the body and maintain youthful vitality.

The fountain of youth has been right under our noses all this time. While it may seem too good to be true, all the effects described above are real and achievable no matter what our age. While it's impossible to live forever, we can delay losing our physical abilities. The muscle-building and hormone-producing effects of weight-training exercise hold the true potential to halt the aging process. The fountain of youth does exist—in the free-weight section of your gym.

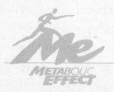

CHAPTER SEVEN

THE METABOLIC EFFECT AND YOUR LIFESTYLE CHOICES

You now have all the nutritional and fitness tools you need to achieve the Metabolic Effect, so it's important to understand how other factors affect your body's fat-burning abilities.

The body's hormonal software is strongly affected by environmental factors such as light, sleep, caffeine, alcohol, hydration, and stress, as well as diet and exercise. Although you may not yet appreciate the role these things play in generating your Metabolic Effect, they are potent hormonal stimulators. Your choices regarding these factors are just as important as your decisions about food and exercise. If you neglect these important aspects of hormonal balance, the Metabolic Effect will be difficult to attain.

Starting when you wake up in the morning, how much attention do you actually pay to these decisions? Like most people, you probably don't think twice about them. In fact, you may not even realize you are making choices that affect every aspect of your physiology every single minute.

Have you ever wondered why some people never seem to make health and fitness progress no matter how well they eat or how much they exercise? That's because in our culture we rarely deal with the other areas affecting health and fitness.

We explain in the following pages why living in a more conscious manner will enhance the hormonal software responsible for the way your body performs. Once you understand how to incorporate quality habits into your lifestyle, you'll find that burning fat, keeping it off, and improving your health are much easier than you ever thought.

THE LIGHT OF DAY

You may be tired of our continued references to historic man and your connection to his ancient physiology, but that is the only way to understand what happened to our culture's collective health and how human physiology actually functions. As a species we are not designed to eat sugar-enriched and salty processed foods or sit behind a computer desk for 8 hours a day.

Look around you. What time of the day is it? Is the sun shining? Is it dark? Besides traveling to the office, gym, or school, did you spend any time today outside in the sunlight? We ask these questions to get you to think about the effects natural light has on your physiology. Before compasses, clocks, and calendars, day changing to night and back again was how people set their sleep/wake cycles. When the sun came up, it was time to work. When the sun went down, it was time to sleep. When the days were shorter, people knew it was winter. When the days were longer, they knew it was summer. They used the position of the sun to know what time of day it was.

Natural light has a tremendous effect on our physiology. What you may not realize is that even a single photon of light hitting your skin can have an effect on your hormones. So imagine the positive effect of rays of light streaming into your bedroom each morning. As light hits your eyes in the morning, the brain and other parts of the body receive messages that say it's time to get up. These messages cause a cascade of hormonal software to begin processing and carrying the commands to rise. In turn, these hormones raise blood sugar, increase heart rate, elevate body temperature, and begin preparing the body for movement.

Cortisol, adrenaline, and other hormones are slowly elevated as day breaks, until they hit a level that gets you up and moving. By the same token, hormones like melatonin, important in the regulation of circadian rhythms, are suppressed by cortisol during the day, but begin to rise at night as cortisol levels drop. Part of this drop in cortisol and other stress hormones occurs due to decreasing light as evening approaches. As a natural response, our hormones evolved to respond to many inputs. Light is the most primal of these inputs.

Now think about what you do at night when the sun goes down. Like most people you probably sit in front of the TV or relax in a lamp-lit room long into the night. Believe it or not, your physiology does not distinguish between the sun, light from a lightbulb, and your computer or television. As far as your metabolism is concerned, if the sun is up you are suppose to be awake and if you are awake you should probably be looking for food. How many people do you know who go home at night, sit down in front of the TV, and then feel themselves drawn to the refrigerator? There they are with artificial sunlight shining on them and their bodies and hormones are asking, "Hey, where's my food?"

Being exposed to light at night may seem benign, but it has a dramatic impact on how your body functions. The processes of life are dualistic and diphasic. This means everything has its opposite, and balance is achieved by the constant interplay between the two "opposing" forces. In Traditional Chinese Medicine (TCM) this concept is called yin and yang. This universal symbol illustrates the connectedness of opposites; there can be no light without dark, no summer without winter, and no hot without cold.

In order to have balance, you must first choose balance in all the relevant aspects of your life, and when it comes to hormones and the Metabolic Effect, balance is everything. When you go back to your understanding of the natural effects of the seasons on your ancient physiology, you will quickly see that summer must lead into winter, which must lead into spring. If this doesn't happen, you'll be unable to achieve the natural balance your physiology seeks.

The pursuit of hormonal balance and the Metabolic Effect is what the body strives for. The body has its own intelligence and knows what it needs to survive. It will innately strive for optimal health and fitness. This makes your job easier. All you have to do is identify and correct the less than ideal lifestyle choices you make. If you choose the standard American lifestyle of high-sugar, high-calorie foods, little activity, and constant exposure to light, you will never regain balance. Where to start? With sleep.

SLEEP: YOUR HORMONAL RESET BUTTON

When was the last time you had a genuinely good night's sleep? The real question is, when was the last time you burned fat, regenerated your cells, and slowed your aging while sleeping?

How and when you sleep is one of the most powerful lifestyle choices you can make. It has been proved in study after study that people who sleep well—quality and quantity—are thinner, happier, more energetic, and healthier than those who toss and turn and don't get a full night's rest.

Sleep is like a hormonal reset button for the body. When you catch a cold, when you're recuperating from surgery, or when your muscles are fatigued or sore from physical labor or a tough workout, sleep is one of the many factors that helps the body heal and gets you on your feet again. Sleep has this effect because it so drastically changes and balances your hormones.

If you're like most people, you have high amounts of cortisol and insulin playing the game of blood-sugar regulation, and leptin rising with each calorie-rich, carbohydrate-dense meal. When you are awake it's hormonal summertime, and if you haven't reached metabolic resistance yet, you're headed there.

Sleep resets the body's hormones for balance. Before electricity allowed us to have light 24 hours a day, the only choice humans had during the cold, dark winter months was sleep, often up to 14 hours a day.

Staying up late watching TV elevates cortisol levels and stress hormones, which you now know raise blood sugar and force insulin to be released to lower it. Over time this interplay leads to metabolic resistance, meaning that the same amount of hormone no longer has the intended effect. Therefore, the body releases more and more of these hormones to accomplish its metabolic agenda. This creates a vicious cycle of carbohydrate cravings and elevated insulin and cortisol, resulting in obesity, early aging, and disease.

Do you want a lean, healthy body or do you want to watch late-night television? If you no longer go to sleep at a reasonable hour, it's because you've made poor choices for so long you now think that is just the way you are. ("I'm a late-night person. I can't fall asleep until one A.M.") It's only the way you are, but you chose to be that way. The good news is that you can also choose *not* to be that way.

Sleep lowers leptin, insulin, and cortisol levels and elevates melatonin, HGH, testosterone, and other hormones. Sleep improves mood, burns fat, and slows the aging process. Sleep is the ultimate antiaging, muscle-building, fat-burning, and mood-enhancing process the body has available to it. If you choose to go to bed late at night because you want to watch a favorite TV show, then your hormonal software will think it's summertime and you will gain weight, and become tired and depressed as you prepare for winter. If you can't miss your favorite late-night show, record it and watch it the next day at an earlier time.

Sleeping for the Metabolic Effect

Eight hours of uninterrupted sleep at night is the minimum amount required for hormonal balance. Sleep quantity is one of the most important considerations in balancing hormones. Every night your body goes through its rhythm of hormonal computing to repair, regenerate, and revitalize the tissues of the body. This process is complicated and takes time.

We compare getting enough sleep to downloading a new piece of computer software. Things happen in sequence and are done a very specific way so that the software will function correctly the next time the computer is turned on. Notice how every time you download new software, you have to restart the computer. If the process is interrupted in some way, what happens? You have to reboot and start again. If something really goes wrong, the computer may lock up, or not function again until the situation is remedied. This is similar to what happens in your body without proper sleep.

Give yourself plenty of time for your body's hormonal software to download and complete its functions. As the hours pass when you are asleep, all the fat-storing hormonal machinery is turned down. Leptin, cortisol, insulin, and adrenaline are lowered, allowing the body to be able to hear the signals of these hormones once again. While that is happening, glucagon, HGH, testosterone, and other growth-promoting and antioxidant hormones like melatonin are elevated.

The combination of this hormonal environment puts you in a fat-burning, antiaging, growth state. This process, however, takes time while the body slowly switches from fat storing to fat burning. The longer you sleep, the more likely you are to make that switch and enjoy several hours of fat burning. People who sleep fewer than 8 hours a night may never reach fat-burning mode at all. For the most effective sleep, 9 hours is closer to ideal.

While many people (especially muscle burners and sugar burners) brag that they function well on just 4 to 6 hours of sleep each night, they are unknowingly damaging their physiology. Over time the body will develop the look of a "stressed-out" physiology. With muscle burners, their arms and legs become thin, loose, and saggy and fat deposits occur around the midsection, a sure sign of elevated stress hormones without the opposing action of growth hormones like HGH and testosterone that sleep raises so well. Muscle burners may feel and look good for a few years on small amounts of sleep, but soon the lean physiques of their younger years give way to a sagging physiology. When sugar burners attempt to get by on just 4 to 6 hours of sleep, constant cravings and hunger set in. Food is always on their minds.

Sleep deprivation is one of the most insidious blocks to achieving the Metabolic Effect. Some people claim that their slowing metabolism or less than youthful appearance is based entirely on the natural consequences of aging, but much of that aging is magnified and accelerated by depriving your body of one of its most essential fat-burning and antiaging commodities—sleep.

HEAD TO BED AT TEN P.M.

The natural rhythm of the sleep cycle is also related to time. Remember, light is what stimulates the hormones that get you up in the morning. If there's light at night, it's more difficult for your hormones to help you sleep. Some people are more susceptible to this than others.

Your ancient physiology is programmed to go to bed shortly after the sun sets in the evening. Artificial lighting, TV, and computer screens circumvent this response by lengthening the time your hormonal-wake software is active. What this means is that the longer you are exposed to light after the sun has gone down, the more you push back your hormonal sleeping software.

Remember, part of your sleeping software includes fat-burning and antiaging hormones like HGH, glucagon, and testosterone. As soon as light comes up again the next morning, that software is shut off, which means that if you sleep 8 hours but go to bed at midnight, only 5 or so hours of that sleep is in the dark. That is not enough time to reset your hormonal software. Studies show that people who go to bed closer to midnight have higher cortisol levels in the morning than those who go to bed around ten P.M. This holds true even when both groups of people sleep for the same number of hours. In order to ensure that your hormonal systems are working for you, the time you go to bed is just as important as how long you sleep.

There are several things you can do to retrain yourself to get to bed earlier. Start by waking up 2 to 3 hours earlier than you usually do for several days to reset your body's circadian physiology. Avoid stimulants, both chemical (coffee, tea, and soda with caffeine) and sensory (bright lights, TV, and loud music), in the evening. A glass of wine or a cocktail may put you to sleep, but alcohol disrupts natural sleep cycles and often does more harm than good.

Muscle burners can benefit from relaxing herbal teas containing chamomile, lemon balm, or passionflower. Sugar burners can drink these beverages and should also eat dinners and snacks that are heavy on protein and light on starch at the end of the day. By going to bed 15 to 20 minutes earlier each evening, mixed burners can adjust their sleep patterns.

TURN OFF THE LIGHTS

Depending on your genetic, metabolic, and psychospiritual sensitivities, even plug-in night-lights and glow-in-the-dark alarm clocks have an effect on sleep. We tell clients—most often muscle burners—who have difficulty falling asleep that moving their alarm clocks away from the bed will increase sleep quality or quantity.

There are things you can do to minimize the effects light has once the sun goes down:

- Dimmers allow enough light so that you can see, but do not create the artificial brightness of full-strength 100-watt lightbulbs. As far as TV and computers are concerned, see if they too are equipped with dimmers. If not, and you have difficulty getting proper sleep, as we've mentioned, their use at night should be limited or avoided. Your best bet is to shut your computer or TV off 1 to 2 hours before bedtime. Reading, taking a relaxing bath, or going for a relaxing evening walk are other beneficial options.
- Candles create an effect similar to dimmers. Candles can be lit several hours before bed. A nice cup of chamomile tea and

a good book read by candlelight are soothing and induce sleep. By using dimmers and candles, you can help your physiology interpret moonlight instead of sunlight.

By reducing your exposure to bright lights after the sun has declined, you will reduce sugar cravings, improve sleep, and help lower your cortisol levels. This allows you to burn fat and regenerates your body at night the way you were designed to.

○ ○ ○

The Night Shift

Health-care professionals, cabdrivers, factory and protective-services workers, and others who sleep during the day can take steps to create the natural effects of night. Darken the room as much as possible with shades and curtains to simulate nighttime. When sleeping, turn off phones, insulate the room from outside noises, and do your best to avoid any interruptions in sleep. Air purifiers or white-noise simulators can be helpful. For those who work at night, a 10- to 30-minute nap during a night shift, if possible, has been shown to increase productivity and blunt some of the negative effects.

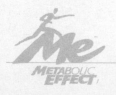

DON'T EAT FOR 2 TO 3 HOURS BEFORE BEDTIME

One of the reasons sleep is so effective at rebuilding the body, burning fat, and slowing the aging process is that it is one of the only times the body has nothing else to do. Think about this: when you eat it can take hours for the food to be digested and assimilated. While proper nutrition is necessary and beneficial, your body also needs time without food. Remember the yin and yang of the natural world? Sleep provides the opposite to the digestion of food and frees resources for regeneration.

If you find it difficult to sleep properly, you need to simulate sleep's effect by avoiding food at night. Sleep is incompatible with eating, which is why it is so beneficial. Adequate sleep quality and quantity allows the perfect situation for lasting fat loss: lower calories and hormonal balance. One of the most effective strategies we see for fat loss with our clients is that they avoid food for 10 to 12 hours at night. For most people that will mean the last meal of the day is between seven and eight P.M. The avoidance of food once the sun goes down will help reverse the hormone resistance of cortisol, insulin, and leptin. There are conditions, such as diabetes and when taking certain medicines, that require you to eat before bedtime or in the middle of the night. In such cases, follow your physician's instructions.

What if you can't go to bed early enough to take full advantage of sleep's effects? After all, life wouldn't be much fun if we just went home, ate an early dinner, and crawled into bed every night. Children, work, or a classic movie on TV all mean a regular bedtime isn't always possible. Go out and see your friends and family, but try to stick to a schedule as much as possible. To make up for any missed sleep, pay close attention to your diet and exercise and employ some relaxation techniques such as meditation, yoga, and tai chi. A 10-minute nap, 5 minutes of deep breathing, or a nice slow walk in the park are relaxing and help blunt some of the negative effects of sleep deprivation.

TAKE A NAP

Napping is a powerful tool in your arsenal for hormonal balance. After a poor night's sleep, cortisol and insulin levels will be elevated—a bad hormonal combination that leads to energy lows, increased hunger, and a constant desire for high-fat, high-sugar foods and stimulating beverages like coffee. It's like having the hard drive crash on your computer. Even if you get the computer started again, it just doesn't seem to run as quickly as it once did.

Taking a 30-minute power nap or a longer 2-hour snooze in the early afternoon allows you to briefly reset your hormonal software by lowering cortisol and normalizing insulin levels. As a result, hunger is controlled, cravings dissipate, and you feel energized.

A 2-hour nap every once in a while is ideal because there's enough time for the brain and body to go through all the important sleep cycles, but even shorter naps of 20 minutes to 1 hour are beneficial when it comes to balancing hormonal fat burning. Naps, however, don't make up for a good night's sleep, but for those with sleep deprivation—infants who need to be fed, sick children, or medications taken during the night—naps help counter the negative hormonal effects keeping you from burning fat.

CONTROL STRESS

Life is stressful. What if you could eliminate some or all of that stress? What if you could go back and redo today over? What if you slept for 8 or 9 hours and woke before the alarm clock went off? Then you did a stimulating workout of just the right intensity for you. What if everything you ate today was perfectly suited to your individual biochemistry? What if when you woke up you made a conscious choice to live the day in total happiness and joy?

If this day really took place, would you be less stressed or more stressed? It's a no-brainer, right? Of course you would feel less stressed, but why? Because during your day you chose to exert influence over the areas of stress you could control.

There is stress that you can control and stress that you can't. We call the total amount of both the controllable stress and the uncontrollable stress you encounter in a day your daily stress load. As your daily stress load increases, your health, mood, energy, productivity, and well-being suffer. The feelings, sensations, and negative associations you feel from stress are directly related to the hormonal software stress puts in motion. Increased heart rate, respiration, sweaty palms, digestive discomfort, headache, difficult vision, and emotional upset all manifest themselves in a particular hormonal environment.

Historic man was under stress too: finding food, seeking shelter, avoiding predators, fending off intruders and famine, and dealing with changing weather were all part of his daily life. Stress, however, did not affect him as it affects us because he slept long, exercised hard, and was forced to stay in the moment.

The best way to deal with stress is to use the tools you have already learned. Get to the gym to offset the high stress hormones and couple them with exertion the way nature intended. Eat healthy, nourishing food. Use your hormonal reset button—sleep—and most important, make a conscious choice to accept stress as a part of life so that you can better anticipate and react to stress in a healthy way. Stress is not the cause of the problem, it is merely a symptom of the world in which we live and the choices we make. Your choices about the proper way to live will allow you to control the stress in your life better rather than having it control you. If you are living the Metabolic Effect lifestyle, your daily stressors will be perceived as less threatening. If stress has less of a negative influence on you, then fat burning becomes much easier.

ALCOHOL

You have probably heard or read that certain alcoholic beverages— red wine, vodka, and dark beers—are good for you in moderation. But just what does "moderation" mean? Excessive alcohol consumption is known to cause dehydration, compromise liver function, and impair brain function. Another little known fact is that alcohol shuts down fat burning and blunts the metabolic effect. In order to understand whether or not alcohol is an appropriate choice for you, you need to define your goals as well as your personal reaction to alcoholic beverages.

Most people who follow health- and fitness-related issues are probably aware of some of the beneficial effects of alcohol. Most experts agree that part of the French paradox—the fact that the French consume a fatty diet and enjoy sweets yet do not suffer the same degree of health issues as other Western people—is due to the consumption of red wine. The Mediterranean diet is also rich in red wine consumption. It is true that resveratrol, a phytonutrient found in grapes and red wine, is being shown to be a very powerful antiaging compound. This compound has the ability to alter many different genetic and metabolic parameters in the body and provide much benefit.

But with the consumption of resveratrol comes the consumption of alcohol. At some point the detrimental effects of the alcohol outweigh the beneficial effects of resveratrol. When trying to understand complex health issues, you have to continuously weigh the risks and the benefits of your choices. This holds true for other alcoholic beverages as well. Often a healthy diet doesn't equal a fat-loss diet. A fat-loss diet, however, is almost always a healthy diet. It's a good idea to remember this when it comes to alcohol. While red wine in moderation can be healthy, it will not aid your fat-loss goals. Save your cocktails and wine for your once-a-week Reward Meal.

Let's take a look at alcohol's metabolic effects in the body. When absorbed in the body, alcohol is broken down into a compound called acetate. When you burn fat, you also produce acetate, which is used in cellular energy production. Excess acetate from alcohol tells the body it doesn't need to burn fat, thus slowing fat burning for several hours. Add to this the dehydrating effects alcohol has and you create a double whammy of slowed fat burning. We've worked with many people who followed their program to the letter, except when it came to drinking alcohol. As a result, their bodies have difficulty sustaining the Metabolic Effect.

If you can't live without a few sips of burgundy at your evening meal, then treat wine or any other alcoholic drink as you would starch. Depending on your metabolic type, you know how many bites of starch you can eat at each meal. Drink your wine, beer, or cocktail in place of your allotted starch bites and enjoy it with food at just 1 meal a day. If you're a sugar burner who usually consumes 5 bites of starch at a meal, then take 5 sips of a nice merlot with your steak and broccoli as long as you forgo the 5 bites of baked potato. For some, however, even this will be too much. Paying close attention to how alcohol affects your biofeedback parameters of energy, hunger, and cravings will give you an idea about your individual tolerance. Sleep is also a useful biofeedback tool when determining how much alcohol you can drink. If alcohol interferes with sleep (you wake up in the middle of the night, for instance), then it's clear that drinking alcohol is interfering with your fat-burning mechanism.

CHAPTER EIGHT

THE ME FOOD PLAN AND MUSCLE-BUILDING RECIPES

We've learned from working with thousands of clients that the key to following the ME Food Plan is to keep it simple and limit your choices. The more variety you introduce, the more likely you are to struggle with the program. If there are no cookies in the pantry, you won't be tempted to eat them. Don't forget, you have your once-a-week Reward Meal when you can eat and drink anything you want!

The first suggestion for limiting your choices has to do with your weekly grocery shopping. Make a list of what you will need for the week and purchase only those items. The majority of our clients prefer not to spend a lot of time shopping and prepping, but if you like fresh, rather than frozen, fruits and vegetables, then feel free to buy red peppers, broccoli, and other items in the produce section. This is just an example of what a shopping list might look like. Create your own list of fat-burning foods you enjoy.

- 12 apples
- 3 pounds ground turkey or bison
- 4 cartons egg whites
- celery
- 1 carton eggs

- 2 rotisserie chickens
- 1 package romaine hearts
- 4 bags frozen mixed vegetables
- 4 baking potatoes or sweet potatoes
- 1 box oat-bran hot cereal
- 1 bag dry-roasted almonds
- 1 box protein bars
- 1 can whey protein powder
- 1 large onion
- 1 head garlic
- 2 jars salsa
- 3 bags frozen blueberries
- 1 jar peanut butter
- 1 box organic cocoa powder
- green tea
- grated Parmesan cheese
- balsamic vinegar
- extra virgin olive oil
- vegetable oil spray

Bring your list with you when shopping to ensure that you buy the right foods for fat burning.

The apples, almonds, protein bars, eggs (hard-boiled), and whey protein powder for smoothies are handy snacks and quick meals. Put your snacks everywhere you might need them—in your gym bag, your car, and your desk at work. The list also includes cocoa powder and peanut butter to help with the munchies and cravings. For major meals, there are egg whites, oat-bran hot cereal and blueberries, and green tea for breakfast.

Everything on the list is there for a reason; there are no extra or "gourmet" ingredients. Ninety-nine percent of our clients tell us that cooking takes too much time, so we focus on meals that take little time to prepare.

Looking at the list, you probably asked, "Hey where's the diet soda, the gallon of milk, and the two loaves of bread?" They're not there because they won't help with your fat-loss goals. If you eat them, you'll send the wrong hormonal signals to your body.

Use the keep-it-simple philosophy when grocery shopping. For the most part, all grocery stores are set up in the same way, with produce, meats, and eggs on the periphery, so stick to those areas. Avoid temptation and don't venture into the aisles packed with processed foods. Always go shopping after you've eaten or you'll be tempted to buy things that don't serve your fat-loss goals.

If you eat most of your meals at home, then buy fresh vegetables and steam, microwave, or roast them. If you're someone who dines out several times a week, buy frozen vegetables because they keep longer.

BE PREPARED

Keeping it simple when it comes to your food choices also includes preparing ahead for the coming week. Our clients who take these steps are our most successful ones. Those who don't plan ahead when it comes to food shopping and advance preparation are the ones who struggle. When you do your grocery shopping, take another hour or two to prepare for the coming week. Cut up the rotisserie chickens when you bring them home and store them in the refrigerator so you can put together a salad at a moment's notice. Wash and thoroughly dry the salad greens. When you want a salad, grab three handfuls of greens and sprinkle on some Parmesan cheese and balsamic vinaigrette. Boil the eggs. Bake the potatoes. Make some chili with ground turkey, onion, garlic, and salsa. Stash everything in storage containers. When you open the fridge, you'll have plenty of choices and won't have to think about what to cook at the last minute. All you have to do for a meal is heat up the potato and chili and steam some vegetables. Taking the few hours to do this will benefit you throughout the week.

REMEMBER TO EAT BEFORE YOU GET HUNGRY

After a long day at the office or with the kids, even 10 minutes seems like a long time to prepare a meal when you're tired and starving. Times like these are when bad choices are made. You're so hungry you'll eat anything, so planning ahead is crucial to avoid snacking on and eating the wrong foods. Most people, if they eat 3 meals a day, eat breakfast, lunch, and dinner, but on our program that allows too much time to pass between meals. As you're now aware, if you don't eat frequently your hunger and cravings will win. In addition to your big meals, you also need to eat something midmorning, midafternnoon, and late afternoon. Proponents of calorie-counting diets believe this is a no-no since between-meal eating adds extra calories. Nothing could be further from the truth. As you've learned, hormones—not the food itself—control what calories you burn. Missing your preemptive snacks leads to overeating and a desire for high-fat, high-sugar, and high-salt foods. Have a protein shake, protein bar, or an apple with a handful of almonds at snack time. You'll eat less food overall, make wise choices, and those calories will take care of themselves.

EATING OUT

When it comes to eating out, again keep it simple and use the tools of visualization and planning. In other words, think ahead and limit the times you're caught unaware or find yourself in a place that doesn't offer the kind of food you want and need. Familiarize yourself with two or three restaurants where you know you can order foods based on their hormonal fat-burning potential. At a Chinese restaurant, skip the rice and noodles and order steamed vegetables with chicken or shrimp. Any restaurant should be glad to accommodate your wishes; after all, you're paying for your food. Being a regular customer helps, but if the establishment won't make changes or substitutions, then don't patronize the place.

PRACTICE MAKES PERFECT

As a result of relying on the calorie-counting model, people often develop, an all-or-none mentality when it comes to food. If you "cheat" or go off your program, don't skip your next meal or try to compensate by eating less. This makes the bad hormonal situation created at the last meal worse. By eating your next snack or meal on schedule, you can restore balance to your fat burning much faster. Cutting back on the amount of food you eat sets hormonal biochemistry into action, resulting in unfavorable changes in hunger hormones, a rise in stress hormones, and cravings for high-calorie foods. Your body is responding as it is designed to. By cutting back on the amount of food you eat, your metabolism slows down and certain hormones are triggered, which results in overeating. Relying on willpower just won't work. No matter what, you'll only last so long before breaking down and eating whatever is in sight. If you choose to change your body by decreasing the number of calories you consume rather than what kind of foods you eat, you're doomed to fail. You'll lose much-needed muscle while on the diet, and regain unnecessary fat when you go off it. We can't stress this enough, but the calorie-counting model of weight loss works against the natural physiology of your body. Remember, you are always only one meal, one exercise session, or one night's sleep away from restoring hormonal balance and fat burning.

With the Metabolic Effect, once you start to eat to balance, trigger, and control the hormones responsible for hunger, cravings, and energy, you will automatically eat fewer calories without even trying. The typical American breakfast of cereal, toast, and orange juice contains more calories and is ultimately less satisfying than the more hormonally balanced breakfast of a 6-egg-white omelet, ¼ cup oatmeal, and ½ cup blueberries. Focusing on meals that have higher amounts of protein and fiber and lower amounts of sugar and fat, and eating those meals more frequently, ensures that you'll be able to resists the all-or-none hormonal influences of low-calorie diets.

TEN TIPS FOR EATING THE METABOLIC EFFECT WAY

1. **Eat 4 to 6 small meals per day.** The fewer meals you eat, the less your body will want to burn fat. The goal is to increase the amount/volume of food you eat during the day without increasing the number of calories. To do so, eat foods with high water, fiber, and protein content. Research shows that people tend to consume the same volume of food every day regardless of calories. High-volume foods satisfy the body through the release of hunger hormones and produce less caloric intake.

2. **Do not eat after eight P.M. or eat only protein after this time.** Sleep can be prime fat-burning time or prime fat-storing time. To burn, rather than store, fat at night, get adequate sleep. Sleep helps to release human growth hormone (HGH), which is a powerful fat-burning and muscle-building hormone. High blood sugar at night has been shown to decrease nighttime HGH. Therefore, going to bed on an empty stomach or only consuming protein before bed is a good fat-burning strategy. Many people eat sugar within a few hours of going to bed and shut off their fat-burning potential at night.

3. **Use the bite rule for starches and sugars.** Insulin is a fat-storing and fat-locking hormone, which means when it is around, calories will be stored as fat and fat can't be used as energy. The major trigger for insulin release is starchy foods and sugar, like bread, pasta, potatoes, cookies, crackers, rice, etc. The body will do best with a small amount of starch/sugar, but excess intake will increase fat storing. By limiting the amount of starch/sugar you consume to bites, you will be able to control insulin levels simply and effectively while avoiding drops in blood sugar that can cause cravings and low energy. In general, most people will want to limit starch/sugar intake to

3 to 15 bites (see page 45) at a meal depending on how insulin sensitive they are.

4. **Eat the right fats.** Certain fats found in foods help burn fat for several reasons. Fat helps control hunger through the release of a hunger hormone called CCK. Certain fats, like omega-3 from fish and grass-fed animals, can turn on fat-burning genes by interacting with cell receptors called PPARs. Your body needs certain fats to burn fat, so don't avoid them completely. Eat fish, nuts, seeds, avocados, olive oil, and grass-fed meat to get the right kinds of fats in your diet.

5. **Eat lean protein at every meal.** Protein is beneficial to fat burning in a number of ways. Protein releases the fat-burning hormone glucagon, which directly opposes the action of insulin and helps burn fat. Protein takes longer for the body to digest than other foods and requires the body to work in order to break it down, which increases the number of calories and heat the body uses. Protein satisfies hunger, helps us stay full, and maintains blood sugar levels to avoid drops in energy. Extra protein also helps build and maintain muscle, which is the body's most important metabolic tissue. The surest way to create cravings and feel deprived is to skimp on protein. Eat your fish, egg whites, chicken, seafood, and meat or use a protein supplement if you're a vegetarian.

6. **Eat protein bars and shakes for quick meals.** Protein bars and shakes (smoothies) are handy foods that can quickly interfere with cravings and hunger. Eat them as small snacks between meals to decrease hunger, provide building blocks for muscle, and stabilize energy. Purchase bars and shakes only if they fit the next rule—the ME label rule.

7. **Learn the ME label rules (page 119).** Packaged foods are difficult to decipher, but the one question to ask is, "Will they make you store fat or burn it?" If you subtract the fiber and protein from the total carbohydrates on a label, the total should be between 5 to 15 or less depending on the type of burner you are. The lower the number, the better. The fat content should be less than 15 and the sodium content less than 200. If not, put it back on the shelf.

8. **Avoid foods that increase hunger and cravings.** Coffee, synthetic sweeteners, and sweet snack foods make you hungry because of their effect on stress hormones and insulin. Instead, choose water, green tea, cocoa, protein, and fiber (vegetables and fruit) instead.

9. **Always eat breakfast.** When you awake in the morning, the body secretes stress hormones to get you going, and breakfast helps regulate this response. If you skip breakfast, these stress hormones will only sustain you for so long before they send you into a ravenous search for food. Ironically, those who say they are never hungry in the morning most likely have an increased stress response and will benefit the most from eating breakfast. Don't skip breakfast or you'll find yourself on a roller-coaster ride of cravings, hunger, and dips in energy throughout the day. Skipping breakfast can lead to eating late at night.

10. **Never let yourself get hungry.** The only time you should feel hungry is when you wake up in the morning. The hunger urge is a powerful subconscious drive. Once you let yourself get hungry, all bets are off. Eat something for your metabolic type every 2 to 4 hours. Eating before you become ravenous will help balance your hormones and elevate your metabolism.

MAINTAINING THE METABOLIC EFFECT

Think about food, exercise, and optimal body composition like elite athletes do. Top-level athletes have everything scheduled and planned out for days, weeks, and months in advance. Everything these athletes do—from the timing of their meals to what they eat to their training regimens to when and how much they sleep—is planned and practiced ad infinitum until it becomes completely ingrained in the subconscious workings of their minds. Sports psychologists note that the most successful athletes are those who are the most organized and regimented, and have in-season, off-season, and in-game habits that support their mission and sport in every way. Before you say, "Well, they're professional athletes; they get paid to be successful at what they do! I have a job, a family, and a life!" know that our most successful clients are those who plan and stick to their program and succeed in attaining and maintaining fat loss despite all the other responsibilities they have. This is perhaps one of the most important lessons fat-loss seekers need to understand. Achieving fat-loss success and mastery requires the same skill and habits exhibited by successful people in athletics, business, or any other endeavor. Planning, scheduling, and practice guarantee mastery and success in anything.

One of the best ways you can plan ahead is to write out your weekly and daily meal plans. You can write out your meal options with some flexibility. This works well especially for those who feel they want guidance but don't want to eat the same foods every day. Choose three options for each meal and snack. Make one a quick, convenient choice, one that takes a little time to prepare, and one that uses leftovers or eating out. This meal plan has few specifics and provides guidelines with several options, which allows some flexibility yet sets up useful parameters. Notice how the times are specific and that every meal is set up to have at least one convenience item as a preemptive strategy. Also notice how the plan establishes a routine to the eating strategy. Finally, all major meals have the option of cooking and eating whatever you like from the metabolic plate for your type. Here's an example of such a plan:

Meal 1: 7:00 A.M.
Option 1: whey protein smoothie
Option 2: omelet with 6 egg whites, diced tomato, chopped
　　　　　spinach, and a sprinkle of feta cheese; 2 pieces Canadian
　　　　　bacon; ¼ cup slow-cooked oatmeal, steel-cut oats, or
　　　　　oat-bran cereal; ½ apple
Option 3: leftovers, according to your metabolic plate, from the
　　　　　previous night

Meal 2: 10:00 A.M.
Option 1: protein bar
Option 2: handful of almonds and 1 piece of fruit
Option 3: handful of nuts and natural beef jerky

Meal 3: 12:00 P.M.
Option 1: whey protein shake
Option 2: large salad with protein (chicken, turkey, fish) and
　　　　　balsamic vinaigrette
Option 3: dine out following your metabolic plate

Meal 4: 3:00 P.M.
Option 1: celery with 2 to 3 tablespoons of peanut butter
Option 2: handful of nuts and fresh fruit
Option 3: protein bar

Meal 5: 6:00 P.M.
Option 1: meal following your metabolic plate
Option 2: dine out following your metabolic plate
Option 3: whey protein smoothie

Meal 6: 8:00 P.M.
Option 1: blueberries and handful of walnuts
Option 2: fruit and 2 to 3 tablespoons of almond butter
Option 3: protein bar

Some people like to be told exactly what to eat and when to eat it. The following plan provides an exact schedule that doesn't vary from day to day and appeals to those who thrive best on a specific eating plan. This is followed until the menu loses its appeal and certain foods are replaced with others. Instead of having eggs for meal 2, eat oatmeal mixed with whey protein and Canadian bacon on the side. Instead of a salad for lunch, order fajitas without the tortillas at a Mexican restaurant. Switch your menus once a week or every few weeks—whatever will keep you on track. The goals are to keep your meal planning simple by eating the same thing every day for a certain period of time and looking at food as fuel, rather than a reward.

Meal 1: 6:00 A.M.
whey protein shake

Meal 2: 8:00 A.M.
omelet with 6 egg whites, 10 bites oatmeal, 1 apple, 1 cup blueberries

Meal 3: 12:00 P.M.
large mixed salad with grilled chicken and balsamic vinaigrette

Meal 4: 2:00 P.M.
fiber supplement and protein bar

Meal 5: 4:00 P.M.
apple with 2 to 3 tablespoons of almond butter

Meal 6: 7:00 P.M.
chicken burger, 10 bites baked sweet potato, steamed broccoli, steamed asparagus

WHAT HAPPENS IF YOU CHEAT?

We're all human. There are times when you want to eat with friends and family and not worry about eating the right foods. We know you'll be confronted with occasions—parties, weddings, vacations, holidays—when you'll be tempted by and want to enjoy what everyone else is eating. That's okay. But don't make it a habit. The good news is that you're just one meal away from restoring hormonal balance again.

Use it as a learning experience. The more you practice the dietary and exercise principles that balance your hormonal biochemistry, the more proficient you will become and the easier it will get. You'll eventually be able to eat the exact amount of starch your body requires at a meal intuitively without counting bites. Eating out in restaurants will be handled with skill and confidence. You won't find yourself nibbling mindlessly on the wrong foods. Practice leads to mastery of the ME Diet.

FAT-BURNING, MUSCLE-BUILDING RECIPES

Our clients tell us that they love to eat, and many even like to cook, but few have time for preparing complicated meals. With that in mind, we've come up with some simple recipes—blueprints really—that provide the right kind of fat-burning, muscle-building nutrition.

Smoothies

Smoothies are the ideal food for the ME Diet. You can drink them morning, noon, and night, for breakfast or as a snack. They are packed with protein and hydrating, vitamin-rich fruits and vegetables. The combinations are endless. Here are some suggestions, but feel free to make your own using the all-you-can-eat fruit and vegetable guidelines on pages 48-50.

Another tip: if you're going to be making a lot of smoothies, invest in a good-quality blender such as a Vita-Mix or Blendtec. Yes, they're expensive, but they turn ingredients into smoothies or juices in seconds without you having to stop and start the machine.

If using frozen fruit, additional ice isn't necessary. Finally, smoothies are best when fresh; they tend to separate if allowed to sit. If a smoothie does separate before you have a chance to enjoy it, give it another whirl in the blender or cover and shake it up in a glass.

You may want to invest in shaker bottles you can take with you on the go. Protein powder, a fiber supplement, and water combined and given a few good shakes are all you need for a quick fat-burning meal anytime.

We recommend coconut water for smoothies because it is packed with more than 500mg of potassium per serving, making it an ideal food for replenishing electrolytes your body has lost during exercise. Coconut water provides manganese, magnesium, sodium, vitamin C, phosphorous, and calcium. It lends a sweet taste to smoothies, reducing the desire or need for additional sweeteners. Finally, buy pure 100 percent coconut water, not coconut cream or coconut milk except where indicated. Also included are cocoa drinks that fight cravings and stave off hunger. Each delicious drink makes one serving.

BASIC BERRY SMOOTHIE

    8 ounces water or coconut water

    1 cup frozen blueberries, raspberries, or a mixture

    1 to 2 scoops whey protein powder

CHOCOLATE–PEANUT BUTTER SMOOTHIE

    8 ounces water or unsweetened rice or almond milk

    1 to 2 scoops whey protein powder

1 tablespoon peanut butter

1 tablespoon cocoa powder

½ cup ice

CINNAMON-WALNUT SMOOTHIE

8 ounces water or coconut water

1 to 2 scoops whey protein powder

½ cup walnuts

1 teaspoon vanilla extract

½ teaspoon cinnamon

½ cup ice

BROWNIE SMOOTHIE

8 ounces coconut water

1 to 2 scoops whey protein

½ cup walnuts

1½ teaspoons vanilla extract

½ to 1 teaspoon cinnamon

1 tablespoon cocoa powder

½ cup ice

PUMPKIN-PATCH SMOOTHIE

8 ounces water or unsweetened rice or almond milk

1 to 2 scoops whey protein powder

2 to 3 tablespoons canned pumpkin puree, *not* pumpkin pie filling

½ teaspoon cinnamon

⅛ teaspoon nutmeg

1 teaspoon vanilla extract

½ cup ice

FROZEN BERRY-CHERRY SLUSHY

½ cup frozen blueberries

½ cup frozen cherries

1 to 1½ cups coconut water or water

For a slushier smoothie, add a few ice cubes.

FRUIT-BOWL SMOOTHIE

8 ounces water or coconut water

1 to 2 cups frozen blueberries, strawberries, mangoes, peaches, and/or bananas

1 to 2 scoops whey protein powder

COCOLOCO SMOOTHIE

8 ounces coconut water

2 to 4 ounces coconut milk

1 to 2 scoops whey protein powder

1 tablespoon plain or vanilla yogurt (optional)

1 to 2 tablespoons cocoa powder

½ cup ice

AVOCADO-CUCUMBER REFRESHER

8 ounces water or coconut water

1 peeled ripe avocado (use 2, if they are small)

½ cucumber, peeled and seeded

1 scoop whey protein powder

½ cup ice

1 to 2 sprigs fresh parsley (optional)

APPLE-CARROT-CUCUMBER SMOOTHIE

8 ounces water or coconut water

1 scoop whey protein powder

1 carrot, peeled and cut up into pieces

½ apple, peeled and seeded

½ cucumber, peeled

Dash cinnamon or nutmeg

½ cup ice

SWEET POTATO PIE SMOOTHIE

8 ounces water or coconut water

1 scoop whey protein powder

¼ cup pecans or almonds

½ medium sweet potato, baked and peeled

Dash cinnamon

½ cup ice

VIRGIN MARY SMOOTHIE

1 scoop whey protein powder

1 tomato, cut up

1 stalk celery, cut up

Dash Tabasco

½ cup ice

BROCCOLI-SPINACH SMOOTHIE

8 ounces water or coconut water

1 scoop whey protein powder

¼ to ½ cup steamed broccoli

1 to 2 handfuls fresh spinach

½ apple, peeled and cored

½ cup ice

VEGETABLE ZINGER

    1 scoop whey protein powder

    1 tomato, cut up

    ½ red pepper, seeded and cut up

    ½ cucumber, peeled and cut up

    1 scallion, cut up

    1 handful fresh parsley or cilantro

    3 tablespoons lemon juice

    ¼ teaspoon freshly ground black pepper

    Tabasco, to taste

    ½ cup ice

HOT COCOA

Meal-in-a-glass smoothies are refreshing and cooling, but sometimes you need a warm, soothing drink, especially when it's cold outside. Add a dash of cinnamon, cayenne (hot peppers pair well with chocolate), or cardamom.

    1 to 2 heaping tablespoons raw organic cocoa powder

    Unsweetened almond or rice milk, to taste

    1 to 2 teaspoons erythritol or xylitol

Add 1 to 2 heaping tablespoons of the cocoa powder to a mug with 8 ounces of boiling water. Add the almond milk to taste, if desired. Add erythritol to taste, for sweetening. You may also put this drink in the fridge to enjoy cold later.

Breakfast

SPINACH-MUSHROOM OMELET
MAKES I SERVING

Protein-packed egg whites from 4 large eggs equal ½ cup. But why go
to the bother of separating eggs? And what are you going to do with
all those yolks? Make it easy on yourself and buy large containers
of commercially available egg whites. Enjoy omelets hot or at room
temperature. Use any of your favorite vegetables listed on page 48 and
the seasonings of your choosing.

Vegetable oil spray

½ cup sliced mushrooms

1 handful fresh spinach, rinsed but not dried

½ cup egg whites, beaten

Heat a small skillet over medium-high heat. Coat the pan with the
vegetable oil spray. Add the mushrooms and sauté for 3 to 5 minutes.
The mushrooms will give up a lot of water, which will then be
reabsorbed as the mushrooms become crisp and golden. Add the
spinach, stirring until wilted. Add the egg whites and cook until
opaque, then turn with a spatula and cook until done.

Variations: Use ½ cup chopped scallions and leftover steamed broccoli
or other vegetable in place of the mushrooms and spinach. Top with
½ cup tomato salsa and/or 1 ounce goat cheese, low-fat Cheddar, or
other low-fat cheese.

EGG WHITE SCRAMBLE

MAKES 1 SERVING

Vegetable oil spray
¼ cup diced onion
¼ cup diced red or yellow pepper
1 small garlic clove, minced
½ cup egg whites, beaten

Heat a small skillet over medium-high heat. Coat the pan with the vegetable oil spray. Add the onion, pepper, and garlic and sauté until softened, about 4 to 5 minutes. Add the egg whites and cook, stirring constantly with a spatula, to the desired doneness.

TURKEY SCRAMBLE

MAKES 1 SERVING

Vegetable oil spray
1 small garlic clove, minced
5 ounces lean ground turkey
1 cup spinach, rinsed but not dried
½ cup diced tomato or salsa

Heat a small skillet over medium-high heat. Coat the pan with the vegetable spray. Add the garlic and turkey and cook, stirring frequently, about 3 to 5 minutes. Add the spinach and cook until wilted. Toss with the tomato and serve hot.

OAT-BRAN CEREAL IN THE MORNING

We recommend hot oat-bran cereal over oatmeal to our clients because it is so high in fiber—5g per ⅓ cup. Our ideal breakfast is a serving of oat-bran cereal and an egg white omelet, but a scoop of whey protein powder can be added to the cereal if you're in a hurry.

¼ cup oat-bran or other high-fiber hot cereal

Optional additions: 1 scoop whey protein powder, 2 tablespoons chopped nuts, 2 tablespoons ground flaxseed, 2 tablespoons wheat germ, 1 teaspoon erythritol, a dash of cinnamon or nutmeg

Stove top: Combine the oat-bran cereal and 1 cup water in a medium saucepan and bring to a boil. Reduce the heat to low and simmer for 4 to 5 minutes. Stir in the optional additions of your choosing.

Microwave: In a microwavable bowl (not plastic!), combine oat bran with 1 cup water and microwave for 2 minutes. Take the bowl out of the microwave, stir, and microwave again for another 2 minutes. Stir in the optional additions of your choosing.

Breakfast on the Go

There are days when you just don't have time to get out the frying pan and get out the door on time, but you want something more than a smoothie. Here are some quick morning ideas that provide the right kind of nourishment so you're not tempted to take the doughnut-and-coffee route later.

- Toast 1 slice high-fiber bread and top with 2 tablespoons peanut butter, 2 ounces low-fat cheese, or 2 tablespoons nonfat cottage cheese.
- Add ½ cup fresh or frozen berries to 8 ounces 2% or nonfat plain yogurt.
- One cup plain, low-fat kefir blended with 1 scoop whey protein powder and 1 tablespoon sugar-free jam.
- Poached Pears (page 210) or Baked Apples (page 210) made ahead. Accompany with 2 ounces nonfat Cheddar cheese, 2 hard-boiled eggs, or a handful of nuts.

- Roasted or poached and sliced chicken breast or rotisserie chicken with an apple.
- Cook oatmeal or multigrain cereal overnight in a slow cooker. Add 1 scoop whey protein powder or ½ cup cottage cheese and some berries.
- Protein bars.

Salt

Many of the recipes here do not list salt because added sodium can be detrimental to your fat-loss goals and your desire to achieve a lean physique. Sodium causes water retention, thus making you look puffy, and prevents you from seeing the definition of your muscles. Not adding salt to your food goes a long way toward helping you shed pounds of extra water. Your heart will thank you too, as excess sodium raises blood pressure.

That doesn't mean that your food should be bland and tasteless. Use spices (cayenne, pepper, cinnamon, nutmeg, etc.) and fresh herbs (parsley, mint, rosemary, thyme, etc.) to perk up your food. Try the sodium-free seasoning mixes such as the lemon-pepper, Mexican, Italian, and garlic-herb blends that are available. Many of these spices are thermogenic, meaning they increase your metabolism to burn fat and contain healthy antioxidants and antiaging compounds.

Salads

CHEF'S SALAD
MAKES 1 SERVING

Hearts of romaine lettuce have a nice crunchy texture.

2 to 3 hearts of romaine, chopped
6 to 8 cherry tomatoes
4 ounces cooked and sliced chicken or one 5-ounce can of tuna,
packed in water
1 hard-boiled egg, white only
1 to 2 ounces shredded low-fat Cheddar cheese
½ cucumber, chopped
2 to 4 radishes, chopped
1 to 2 tablespoons ME Vinaigrette

Toss all the salad ingredients together and then add the vinaigrette.

SPINACH SALAD
MAKES 1 SERVING

Add the protein of your choosing to this salad.

4 ounces cooked and sliced chicken, pork tenderloin, beef, or
turkey breast
1 to 2 handfuls fresh spinach, well rinsed and dried
¼ red onion, thinly sliced into half-moons
6 to 8 cherry tomatoes
2 tablespoons raw or roasted almonds
Freshly ground black pepper
1 to 2 tablespoons ME Vinaigrette

Toss all the salad ingredients together. Dress with the vinaigrette.

CHICKEN-AVOCADO SALAD
MAKES 2 SERVINGS

This salad, which is rich in glutamine, will help you hold on to the muscles you are building!

2 cups finely chopped green, purple, or napa cabbage
½ avocado, sliced
¼ red onion, diced
2 chicken breasts, cooked and sliced
12 cherry tomatoes
Juice of ½ lemon
2 tablespoons extra virgin olive oil
Freshly ground black pepper
Dash garlic powder, optional, to taste

Toss the cabbage, avocado, red onion, chicken, and tomatoes together in a bowl. Whisk the lemon juice, oil, pepper, and optional garlic powder together in a small bowl. Toss with the salad and enjoy.

◦ ◦ ◦

Salads

Salads become boring when you make them with the same ingredients every day. Avoid the not-another-salad syndrome by using a blend of greens with different colors and textures—Boston lettuce, arugula, finely shredded kale, spinach, radicchio, Belgian endive, romaine, escarole. Wash the greens when you bring them home from the market, dry them well in a salad spinner, and keep refrigerated in a plastic bag. When it comes to fresh sprouts, there are many varieties to choose from—alfalfa, radish, and mung beans.

Add fresh vegetables (grated carrots, thinly sliced scallions, cucumbers, red peppers, tomatoes, radishes) or any leftover roasted vegetables. Sliced apples or pears are also good additions. Four to six ounces of hard-boiled egg whites, chicken, turkey, pork, tuna, salmon, or beef turn a bowl of greens into a main course.

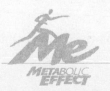

Rotisserie Chicken: Your New Best Friend

Save yourself time and buy a rotisserie chicken at the supermarket once a week. When you get home remove the skin and then separate the meat from the carcass. Cover and store in the refrigerator so you'll have cooked chicken ready for the following dishes.

CHICKEN SALAD
MAKES 1 SERVING

If you don't have chicken on hand, this recipe also tastes great with turkey, lean sliced beef, or a can of tuna.

½ cucumber sliced
½ tomato
Handful sprouts
1 cup chicken
2 cups mixed greens or spinach
1 tablespoon ME Vinaigrette

Toss ingredients together and serve on whole-wheat bread.

CHICKEN BOATS
MAKES 1 SERVING

1 cup shredded chicken
Cherry tomatoes, as many as desired
1 to 2 tablespoons ME Vinaigrette, optional
Romaine lettuce leaves, as many as desired

Mix the chicken, tomatoes, and dressing together in a bowl. Serve on lettuce leaves.

CHICKEN SOUP

MAKES I TO 2 SERVINGS

This recipe is easily doubled or tripled for freezing for meals later in the week.

2 cups low-sodium chicken broth
¼ cup minced onion
¼ cup frozen peas
1 cup shredded chicken
Black pepper
Scallions

Heat the chicken broth in a saucepan over medium heat. Add the onion and frozen peas and bring to a boil. Turn down the heat to medium-low and add the shredded chicken. Simmer for 5 minutes and garnish with the black pepper and scallions before eating.

THAI CHICKEN SOUP

MAKES 2 SERVINGS

This delicious recipe can easily be doubled or tripled.

1 tablespoon olive oil
1 minced garlic clove
1 to 2 tablespoons red or green Thai curry paste (available in the international aisle)
1 tablespoon Thai fish sauce
1 teaspoon erythritol (see page 128)
1 (13.5-oz) can light coconut milk
2 cups low-sodium chicken broth
1 cup snow peas or frozen peas
1 can water-packed bamboo shoots
1 cup mushrooms
½ cup chopped tomatoes
¼ teaspoon crushed red pepper
2 cups shredded chicken
1 to 2 handfuls fresh cilantro
3 handfuls fresh spinach leaves
Lime wedges, for serving

Heat the olive oil and garlic in a saucepan. Sauté the garlic just until it loses its white color. Stir in the Thai curry paste and blend well. Add the Thai fish sauce (nam pla) and erythritol. Add the coconut milk, chicken broth, peas, bamboo shoots, mushrooms, and tomatoes. Sprinkle in the pepper. Bring to a boil and then lower the heat to a simmer. Add the chicken, cilantro, and spinach. Simmer for 3 to 5 minutes. Serve hot, accompanied with lime wedges.

CHICKEN-VEGETABLE WRAP

MAKES 1 SERVING

> 1 cup shredded chicken
> Shredded carrots
> ½ avocado, peeled and sliced
> 1 high-fiber, low-carbohydrate tortilla wrap
> Fresh lemon or lime juice, for serving
> Tahini or olive oil, for serving

Arrange the chicken, some carrots, and the avocado on the tortilla wrap. Squeeze on some fresh lemon or lime juice and drizzle with the tahini or olive oil before rolling up.

METABOLIC EFFECT VINAIGRETTE DRESSING

Some clients tell us that they're eating so many fruits, vegetables, and salads, but not burning fat and losing weight. When we sit down with them and go over their food choices, we often find that they're using excessive amounts of high-fat dressings. We came up with an all-purpose vinaigrette that can be used on fish, chicken, vegetables, and salads, along with some tips for making and using it.

- Use the best-quality ingredients you can afford. A little bit of a special extra virgin olive oil will add more flavor to the dressing than some cheap brand.

- Use cider or balsamic vinegar in place of red wine vinegar for a less acidic taste.

- Lemon juice cuts the vinegary taste.

- Start by drizzling on 1 tablespoon over a salad. Toss and taste to see if you need more. The food should have just a glaze of dressing.

- For a variation, add 1 finely chopped shallot and 1 teaspoon Dijon mustard to the dressing. Chopped fresh herbs can also be added.

- Keep the dressing in the refrigerator in a glass jar and shake well before using.

½ cup cider or balsamic vinegar
2 tablespoons lemon juice
⅓ cup extra virgin olive oil
Mustard, optional
Chopped shallot, optional

Combine the vinegar, lemon juice, and olive oil in a lidded jar. Add the mustard and chopped shallot if desired. Shake well before using.

Main Dishes

QUICK CHILI
MAKES 3 TO 4 SERVINGS

When you want something warm and satisfying, try this chili, which takes less than 30 minutes from start to finish.

1 tablespoon olive oil
1 small onion, diced
2 garlic cloves, minced
1 tablespoon cumin
2 tablespoons chili powder

¼ teaspoon red pepper flakes
1 red pepper, seeded and diced
1 green pepper, seeded and diced
12 to 16 ounces lean ground beef or turkey
1 (28-ounce) can fire-roasted diced tomatoes
Shredded low-fat Cheddar cheese

Heat the olive oil in a large saucepan or Dutch oven. Add the onion
and garlic and sauté until softened, about 5 minutes. Stir in the
cumin, chili powder, and red pepper flakes. Add the peppers and
cook for 5 minutes, until soft. Add the beef and sauté until brown.
Add the tomatoes. Cover and cook over medium-low heat, stirring
occasionally, until the peppers are soft, about 10 to 15 minutes. Ladle
into bowls and serve with 2 tablespoons Cheddar.

QUICK CHICKEN BREASTS

*Having cooked, skinless, boneless chicken breasts in the fridge is
like money in the bank for the Metabolic Effect. You can use them in
salads, wraps, soups, and other dishes. We offer four ways to cook them
and suggest that you make 8 to 10 at a time, so you'll always have some
cooked protein on hand.*

Microwave: Place 2 skinless, boneless chicken breasts on a microwave-
safe plate. Cover with another plate. Microwave on high for 3 minutes,
turn the breasts over, and microwave for 3 more minutes. Season with
your choice of any sodium-free spice blend.

Poached: Place 2 skinless, boneless chicken breasts in a saucepan with
water or low-sodium chicken broth to cover. Bring to a boil, then
immediately lower the heat to a simmer and poach for 4 to 6 minutes.
Allow the chicken breasts to cool in the broth; they will be tender rather
than tough. Season with your choice of any sodium-free spice blend.

Pan-Fried: Heat a large frying pan over medium-high heat. Spray the pan with vegetable oil spray. Season 4 chicken breasts with your choice of seasoning and add to the pan. Cook on one side until the edges become opaque, about 5 to 7 minutes depending on the thickness. Turn, using tongs, and cook until done, about another 5 to 7 minutes.

Stove Top or George Foreman Grill: Place plain or seasoned chicken breasts on the grill and cook until done, about 7 to 9 minutes.

STIR-FRIED BEEF AND BROCCOLI

MAKES I SERVING

This is a basic stir-fry recipe. Substitute chicken, lean pork, or shrimp for beef. Change the vegetables by using bell peppers, onions, bok choy, spinach, snow peas, or watercress in place of or along with the broccoli. If you want to kick up your stir-fry, add a dash of red pepper flakes with the ginger, garlic, and mushrooms.

Vegetable oil spray
1 teaspoon grated fresh ginger
1 garlic clove, finely minced
½ cup chopped button mushrooms
½ cup broccoli florets
2 teaspoons low-sodium soy sauce mixed with 1 tablespoon water
6 ounces lean beef, such as sirloin or round steak, thinly sliced
1 scallion, thinly sliced

Heat a nonstick skillet over high heat and spray with vegetable oil spray. Add the ginger, garlic, and mushrooms and cook, stirring constantly, for 2 minutes. Remove the vegetables to a bowl using a slotted spoon. Add the broccoli to the hot skillet along with the soy sauce and water. Cook for 3 to 4 minutes, stirring constantly, until the broccoli is bright green and tender but not mushy. Add the broccoli to the mushrooms. In the same skillet, cook the beef until done, about 3 minutes, stirring constantly. Add the vegetables to the beef and heat through. Garnish with the scallion and enjoy.

○   ○   ○

What About Soy?

You'll notice that we don't include soy products—tofu and soy milk—in our recipes, which puzzles many of our clients who think soy is a healthy addition to their diets. Soy is not a good idea when it comes to fat loss and hormones. The hormone produced by the thyroid gland is a major metabolic stimulator for fat burning and energy, and the isoflavones (organic compounds) in soy block a key enzyme responsible for the production of the hormone. This may be especially worrisome for those with hypothyroidism.

The same compounds in soy are also known to be phytoestrogens, which means they behave like weaker versions of the estrogen we produce. Estrogen also interrupts thyroid hormone action. In addition, estrogen, including the weaker estrogens in soy, can oppose the action of testosterone, which is one of the body's major muscle-building and fat-burning hormones.

Fermented soy products such as miso, tempeh, and natto have already been "broken down" by their bacteria and enzymes, making their protein and carbohydrate molecules more digestible and less able to interfere with fat burning.

The bottom line is that soy foods can be an impediment to fat loss. While the occasional tofu dish or a bowl of edamame won't adversely affect your fat-burning goals, don't be lured into thinking that soy sausage, soy milk, soy ice cream, soy chips, and other soy products are good for you.

One exception is that vegetarians and vegans will do just fine with some soy protein and other soy foods in their diet, but rice protein, hemp protein, and other alternative protein sources are a much better option.

Vegetables

OVEN FRIES

MAKES 2 TO 4 SERVINGS, DEPENDING ON THE SIZE OF THE POTATO

Potato skins are packed with fiber and nutrients, so just scrub the potatoes well with a brush before cutting up. One serving equals ½ a medium potato.

Vegetable oil spray
1 medium russet potato, unpeeled and cut into ¼-inch sticks
Sodium-free seasoning blend of your choice

Preheat the oven to 400°F. Line a baking sheet with parchment paper or aluminum foil. Spray the baking sheet with vegetable oil spray. Arrange the potatoes on the baking sheet and sprinkle on the seasoning. Bake for 20 to 25 minutes, turning the potatoes every 5 minutes until they are golden and crisp. Serve hot.

BAKED SWEET POTATOES

Preheat the oven to 400°F. Scrub and pierce sweet potatoes in several places with the tines of a fork. Bake for 25 to 35 minutes, until cooked through. And, yes, you can eat the skin on sweet potatoes!

STEAMED SWEET POTATOES

Scrub and slice the sweet potatoes into 1-inch rounds. Place them in a saucepan and cover with water. Bring the water to a boil and cook for 5 to 7 minutes, until the potatoes are tender and the skin starts to separate from the potatoes. These will keep in the refrigerator for several days.

ROASTED SWEET POTATOES

Keep a bowl of these roasted sweet potatoes in the refrigerator.

Preheat the oven to 400°F. Line a baking sheet with aluminum foil or parchment paper. Scrub and slice 2 or more sweet potatoes into 1-inch rounds. Toss the slices in a bowl with 1 tablespoon vegetable oil, freshly ground black pepper, and ¼ to ½ teaspoon cinnamon. Arrange the potatoes on the baking sheet, cover with aluminum foil, and bake for 30 minutes. Remove the pan from the oven and turn the potatoes, using a spatula. Return the pan to the oven and bake for another 20 minutes, until the potatoes are brown and crisp.

ROASTED BRUSSELS SPROUTS AND MUSHROOMS

MAKES 2 TO 4 SERVINGS

Steamed or boiled vegetables are boring. Try roasting them at 400°F and you'll be amazed by how sweet, tender, and tasty they become. Substitute cremini, shiitake caps, or portobellos for the button mushrooms. Instead of sprouts, try broccoli, cauliflower, fennel, green beans, broccoli rabe—just about any firm vegetable will work. If you're lucky enough to have any vegetables left over, puree them the next day with some low-sodium chicken broth for a hearty bowl of soup.

4 cups halved brussels sprouts
2 cups halved button mushrooms
1 garlic clove, minced
Freshly ground black pepper
2 tablespoons extra virgin olive oil

Preheat the oven to 400°F. Toss all the ingredients together in a baking pan, making sure everything is coated with the oil. Roast the vegetables for 15 to 20 minutes, until they're tender but not overcooked. Serve hot or at room temperature.

ROASTED CAULIFLOWER AND LEEK SOUP

MAKES 4 SERVINGS

1 small head cauliflower, trimmed and cut into florets
1 leek, thoroughly washed and sliced into 1-inch rounds
2 garlic cloves, to taste
Dash onion powder
Dash garlic powder
Freshly ground black pepper
2 tablespoons olive oil
2 to 4 cups low-sodium chicken stock

Preheat the oven to 400°F. Toss all ingredients together in a baking pan, making sure everything is coated with the oil. Bake for 20 to 25 minutes, until the cauliflower is tender when pierced with a fork. Put the vegetables into a blender with 1 cup chicken stock, cover, and blend until smooth. Pour the puree into a saucepan and stir in more stock until the soup is the desired consistency. Simmer until heated throughout. Season to taste. Ladle into bowls and enjoy.

Main Dishes

SPICY PORK TENDERLOIN
MAKES 4 SERVINGS

Lean, yet meaty pork tenderloin cooks in no time. Each one weighs about 1 to 1½ pounds, so they cook in 30 minutes or less. You can roast the pork with just a sprinkling of seasoning. Add flavor by marinating them in low-sodium soy sauce and ginger for Asian flavors, or use a low-sodium rub with Moroccan (cinnamon, ginger, coriander, cloves) or Indian (cumin, cardamom, nutmeg, black pepper) spices. Quickly searing or browning in a frying pan before roasting imparts a crisp crust to the meat, but it's not necessary. Finally, take the meat out of the refrigerator about 30 minutes before cooking, if you have time, and let it sit at room temperature.

Vegetable oil spray
One 1- to 1½-pound pork tenderloin, trimmed of any membrane or silver skin
4 scallions, sliced lengthwise
Dash red pepper flakes or cayenne pepper
4 to 6 drops hot chili oil

Preheat the oven to 400°F. (If you want to sear the pork, heat an ovenproof skillet over medium-high heat. Spray the skillet with vegetable oil and sear the tenderloin, turning with tongs, and brown all sides. This shouldn't take more than 3 to 5 minutes. Remove from the heat and add the scallions to the pan. Sprinkle with pepper flakes and drizzle with hot chili oil.) If not searing put the pork in a small roasting pan and sprinkle with pepper flakes and chili oil. Scatter the scallions around the pork. Roast the pork until an instant-read meat thermometer inserted diagonally into the thickest part of the meat registers 155°F. Remove from the oven, cover with foil, and let sit for 5 to 10 minutes before slicing.

CLASSIC BEEF PATTIES

MAKES 6 PATTIES

Use lean ground beef and bake six burgers at one time so you have them on hand. Use lettuce leaves as wrappers instead of burger buns.

2 pounds lean ground beef
1 tablespoon finely minced garlic
Optional seasonings: black pepper, onion powder, or seasoning mix

Preheat the oven to 400°F. Mix the ground beef, garlic, and seasonings in a bowl and divide into 6 portions. With wet hands, flatten the meat into 6 patties. Place them on a ridged broiler pan so the excess fat can drip off. Bake until cooked through, about 10 to 12 minutes, depending on your preference.

Variations: Substitute ground turkey for ground beef. If you're feeling adventurous, ground buffalo is a lean, healthy alternative that is now available in most grocery stores.

CHICKEN FAJITAS

MAKES 2 FAJITAS

Chicken tenderloins, or chicken fingers, are cut from breast meat. You can find these in the poultry section of any supermarket, or cut skinless, boneless chicken breasts into thin strips.

Vegetable oil spray
8 to 10 chicken tenderloins
1 small onion, sliced into thin half-moons
2 cups thinly sliced red, yellow, or orange peppers
2 high-fiber whole-grain tortilla wraps
Dash sodium-free Mexican seasoning

Heat a frying pan over medium-high heat. Spray with vegetable oil. Add the chicken tenderloins and cook on all sides until done, about 5 minutes, and remove to a plate. Add the onion to the pan and sauté the onion until soft, about 5 minutes. Add the peppers to the onion and sauté until the peppers are done but slightly crisp, another 3 to 5 minutes. Divide the chicken and onion-pepper mixture between 2 warm tortillas and sprinkle with the seasoning before eating.

STIR-FRIED BROWN RICE

MAKES I SERVING

Here's a good way to use up leftover brown rice. To make a main-course dish, stir in 4 to 6 ounces leftover cooked chicken, pork tenderloin, or shrimp. Any dark green leafy vegetable can be substituted for the spinach. Of course, this dish can easily be multiplied.

Vegetable oil spray
1 teaspoon minced ginger
2 scallions, diced
1 cup chopped mushrooms
1 to 2 garlic cloves, minced
Handful spinach, well rinsed and chopped
1 cup cooked rice

Heat a frying pan over medium-high heat. Spray with vegetable oil. Add the ginger, scallions, mushrooms, and garlic and sauté until tender, about 3 to 5 minutes. Add the spinach and stir until wilted. Add the rice and stir to incorporate the vegetables. Cook until fragrant, about 2 to 4 minutes.

Desserts

POACHED PEARS
MAKES 2 SERVINGS

Keep poached pears in the fridge to enjoy with oatmeal or an 8-ounce serving of plain nonfat yogurt. Double the recipe if you wish.

2 Bosc pears
2 tablespoons erythritol (see page 128)
Dash cinnamon

With a melon baller, scoop out the core of the pears from the bottom. Slice a small bit of each pear off the bottom so they will stand up. In a saucepan, bring ½ inch of water to a boil, add the erythritol, and stir to dissolve. Lower the heat, place the pears in the saucepan, and sprinkle with cinnamon. Cook, occasionally spooning the syrup over the pears, until they are tender, about 15 minutes.

BAKED APPLES
MAKES 2 SERVINGS

2 apples, such as Cortland, Empire, Fuji, or Gala
¼ cup rolled oats
¼ cup finely chopped walnuts
¼ cup raisins
½ teaspoon cinnamon
¼ teaspoon nutmeg
1 tablespoon erythritol or other sweetener

Preheat the oven to 375°F. Starting at the stem end, push an apple corer through the apple, but leave ½ inch at the bottom to form a "bowl." Turn the corer, scoop out the core, and discard. In a small bowl, combine the oats, walnuts, raisins, cinnamon, nutmeg, and erythritol. Divide the mixture and spoon into the hollowed-out apples. Place the apples in an ovenproof dish with space between them. Bake until the apples are soft but not mushy, about 30 to 35 minutes.

APPLESAUCE
MAKES 6 SERVINGS

Store-bought applesauce is just too sweet. It's so easy to make it fresh, plus it keeps for a week in the refrigerator. Spread some on whole-grain toast or serve as an accompaniment to the Spicy Pork Tenderloin (page 206).

4 apples, such as McIntosh, Gala, or Honey Crisp, peeled, cored, and cut into 1-inch chunks
1 teaspoon cinnamon

Place the apple chunks in a saucepan and cover with water. Bring to a boil, then decrease the heat to medium-low and simmer. Stir occasionally until the apples break down, about 15 minutes. For a creamier applesauce, double or triple the cooking time; just make sure the heat is low so the applesauce doesn't burn. Sprinkle with cinnamon and enjoy!

COCONUT MACAROONS
MAKES 10 TO 12 MACAROONS

A simple cookie to put together when you want something sweet.

1 (8-ounce) package shredded unsweetened coconut
6 egg whites
1 tablespoon vanilla extract
¼ cup erythritol or other sweetener
6 ounces bitter or semisweet chocolate

Preheat the oven to 350°F. Combine the coconut, egg whites, vanilla, and sweetener together in a large mixing bowl. Using wet hands, roll 2 tablespoons of the batter into golf ball–size balls. Arrange the balls on a baking sheet lined with parchment paper. Bake until golden brown, checking frequently so they don't burn, about 12 to 15 minutes. While the cookies are baking, melt the chocolate in a heavy saucepan over low heat. When the coconut balls are done, remove them from the oven and use tongs to transfer to a ceramic plate. Use the tines of a fork to drizzle the chocolate over the macaroons. Chill the macaroons in the refrigerator until the chocolate is set, about an hour. Cover and store extras in the refrigerator.

COCONUT-CHOCOLATE-CHERRY ICE

MAKES 4 SERVINGS

A glass baking dish is preferable because the coating on metal pans can be scraped off along with the frozen ice.

1 (13.5-oz) can coconut milk (Chaokoh or True Thai brands)
1 teaspoon vanilla extract
¼ cup erythritol or other sweetener
½ cup frozen pitted cherries
¼ cup shaved dark chocolate (use a vegetable peeler)

Stir the coconut milk, vanilla, and sweetener together in a 9-by-9-inch glass baking dish, mixing well. Sprinkle the cherries and chocolate over the coconut milk mixture. Cover with plastic wrap and freeze until set, about 2 hours. Spoon into bowls.

METABOLIC EFFECT GELATIN
MAKES 6 TO 8 SERVINGS

Make your own gelatin snack using unsweetened fruit juice and Knox gelatin. It's filling, high in protein, and good for your joints. For additional sweetness, add a natural sweetener like xylitol, if desired.

8 envelopes Knox gelatin
2 cups all-natural unsweetened fruit juice or fruit puree, cold or at room temperature
4 cups all-natural unsweetened fruit puree or berry juices
2 tablespoons natural sweetener, such as XyloSweet, ZSweet, Zero, or Sweet Simplicity, optional

Sprinkle the gelatin over the cool juice in a large bowl and let stand for 1 minute. Bring the remaining 4 cups juice to a boil, and add to the gelatin. Stir until the gelatin dissolves completely. Add sweetener, if desired. Pour the mixture into a rectangular pan.

Refrigerate until firm, about 3 hours, and enjoy as a snack.

CHAPTER NINE
MAKING THE ME DIET WORK FOR YOU

Through the years of helping people make remarkable changes in their bodies with the ME Diet, we discovered the key factors that make a real difference. While metabolic messengers from food and exercise impact how your body looks and feels, they also have a profound effect on your mood, focus, motivation, and thinking, another positive aspect of hormonal fat loss over the caloric-aerobic-weight-loss model.

How you think and feel are also conduits for hormonal change and have an effect on your body. Feelings of sadness make you less motivated, lower your energy, and make you seek out certain foods, while positive feelings such as being in love can do the reverse. You will fully reach the Metabolic Effect when your thoughts and feelings line up with the way your body looks and functions. Bringing the mind and spirit together with the body allows you to make the full transition into fat burning forever: the Metabolic Effect.

THE UNCONSCIOUS VERSUS SUBCONSCIOUS MIND

Your unconscious mind is your automatic nervous system. When you're in a stressful situation, you don't have to think about what to do next: your unconscious takes over. Most people try to control their actions with conscious thoughts because that is what they are aware of, but the real power for change lies in the automatic, instinctual action of the unconscious. This is where cravings for certain foods come from, where our love or disdain for exercise comes from, and where our beliefs and our perceptions about ourselves reside. Once you learn to harness the automatic workings of the body, you can take charge of your choices and exert control over them.

For example, the unconscious mind can process 4 billion bits of information per second. In comparison, your conscious mind can process only 2,000 bits of information per second. To explain this huge difference, think of the processing power of the unconscious mind as the size of the earth, with the conscious mind the size of a single sailboat in the ocean on earth. The differences in magnitude between the two are enormous, which is why attempting to change your behavior through conscious thought is a very poor strategy for success. How can tapping into your unconscious aid in achieving the full metabolic effect?

One of the best ways to use the unconscious mind and harness its power for change is to put your imagination to work. Children are great at this, but as we grow up we often lose our capacity to dream big. Reawakening our imagination, thoughts, beliefs, and emotions can help, rather than sabotage, us. The thing to understand about our unconscious behavior and our brain is that whether we are actually doing something or imagining it, the brain doesn't know the difference. Imagine cutting into a fresh, juicy orange. The fresh juice spills out and you can smell the distinct aroma of citrus. See yourself cutting a perfect wedge of that orange. Now envision picking that wedge up, taking a big bite, and letting the juice run down your chin and hands. Shut your eyes and really imagine this. Is your mouth watering? That's because your unconscious actually believes you just ate an orange. The more details fed into your imagination, the more your unconscious becomes convinced it's true.

Two studies into the imaginations of athletes show just how real this phenomenon is. In the first study, researchers tested the free-throw shooting accuracy in a group of basketball players. They were divided into three groups. Group one was instructed to go to the gym every day and shoot free throws for one hour. Group two was instructed to go to the gym every day, but rather than actually shooting free throws, they were told to visualize shooting free throws. The third group was told to do nothing, to not even think about basketball. At the end of the study, the group that actually shot baskets improved their free-throw percentage by 24 percent. Amazingly, the group that imagined shooting free throws improved their free-throw shooting by 23 percent. The group who did nothing regressed in their percentage.

Follow-up studies compared groups who did both mental imagery and shot baskets to groups who just shot baskets or only imagined shooting baskets. In these studies the group doing both mental imagery and shooting baskets performed the best. These studies demonstrate that your thoughts, your imagination, and your confidence in yourself profoundly impact your success. Every time you take action or imagine yourself completing a task, you're reprogramming your automatic mind toward a different reality. Understand that consciously thinking positive thoughts does not work; the only way change comes is if your unconscious mind believes. And when it does, the changes you can make are startling and powerful.

METABOLIC MESSENGERS AND YOUR METABOLIC TYPE

As we've explained, everyone is treated the same when it comes to the counting-calories and aerobic-exercise weight-loss models. If you don't lose weight or gain it all back following those tried-and-not-true programs, you think of yourself as weak, unable to stick with anything, and undeserving of looking and feeling good.

We want you to understand that the same hormonal messengers that trigger your fat-burning mechanisms also affect your motivation and mood. Doctors frequently prescribe these metabolic molecules in the form of antidepressants or antianxiety medications to help people who suffer from depression or anxiety. Molecules like dopamine, serotonin, GABA, and acetylcholine serve much like the signal traveling through a phone line. The ratios of these neurohormones determines to a large degree how you feel, how motivated you will be to work out, and whether you will crave sugar, salt, or chocolate. These are the messengers of the automatic brain. You now know that exercise and diet can exert influence over these molecules. However, you also should understand that your beliefs are often hardwired into your automatic mind. Often a change in diet and exercise can get the system moving, but in order to make the full switch to the Metabolic Effect, you have to work at behaviors and beliefs. Both action and imagination have a huge influence over these molecules. When you get the diet, exercise, and mental and emotional signals all working together, change becomes much easier than you have ever dreamed.

Interestingly, the type of burner you are has some influence here. Muscle burners tend to be highly goal oriented and driven to take action. They also tend to be people who needlessly worry, take on too many responsibilities, and easily become overwhelmed. They are often so busy that they forget to stop and eat. Sugar burners, on the other hand, feel the same demands, but their response is usually different. They often eat to soothe their nerves, prefer to be couch potatoes, and respond to situations by choosing to do nothing. Mixed burners can go either way, taking on the characteristics of sugar burners or muscle burners depending on lifestyle factors like sleep, drinking caffeine, and food choices. Mixed burners are often pushed in either direction by unconscious beliefs and habits they have developed over time. For instance, a mixed burner who grew up in a family where money was tight may be pushed into a negative pattern of cravings and hunger when he or she is under financial stress. In general, stress moves mixed burners into more of a muscle-burning state while lack of exercise moves them more into a sugar-burning state. Often the demands of their lives combined with established habits and beliefs determine how they function. This allows them to remain balanced, yet makes it harder for them to locate their emotional triggers.

Depending on the metabolic tendencies of an individual, certain tactics for change should be emphasized. We, however, have found that all types respond universally to change when three key aspects are addressed. We call this purpose, focus, and choice, or PFC.

PURPOSE, FOCUS, AND CHOICE: YOUR FORMULA FOR CHANGE

There are many theories as to why people behave and act in a certain way, and there are just as many schools of thought on how to go about changing that behavior for the better. From working with our clients we discovered that there are three key things that make mastering the Metabolic Effect more effective: purpose, focus, and choice, or PFC.

When we sit down with a client who is desperate and has tried everything from starvation fasts to the latest deprivation diets to change the way his body looks, functions, and feels, we do two things. First, we find the underlying hormonal imbalances that have shut down the fat-burning metabolism. Second, we deal with the emotional aspects of long-held thinking and beliefs that impact his ability to make lasting changes, not an easy task because the unconscious mind isn't as open or as transparent as the conscious mind. By tapping into a person's true purpose and his ability to stay focused on his desires, the workings of the automatic nervous system become more apparent. Once he does this, he is able to connect his minute-to-minute choices directly to something bigger and more meaningful and begins to realize the true power of the metabolic change at the level of the mind as well as the body.

Purpose

One of the first questions we ask a new client is, "What is your purpose in coming to us?" When the client looks confused and gives us a blank stare, we know we're in for some serious reworking of his or her unconscious awareness. We want to hear what drives our clients, or what is their greatest desire. Purpose gives us energy, focus, and perseverance during our most trying times. Attempting to make a metabolic shift without knowing the reason you're doing so is like driving to someone's home when you don't have the address. You'd be driving forever without ever reaching your destination. Purpose is what gives you direction and motivation for achievement.

If you have a solid purpose for doing something, making changes will be easier than you thought. But that reason has to be tied to realistic goals. Your true purpose for following the ME Diet will push you to wake early and do your workout, give you the discipline necessary to prepare and stick to the food that's right for your metabolic type, and motivate and sustain you for the long haul.

Allison was a client who loved the feeling of reaching that state of optimal function we call the Metabolic Effect, yet she was unable to sustain it. She often missed workouts and ate several Reward Meals each week, not just one. After one particular session, we asked Allison about her ultimate goal in life and how achieving her peak metabolic function fit into it. At first she struggled to put her thoughts into words, but then said her ultimate goal was to be a source of strength and a role model for her young daughter, who was becoming overweight. In essence, we explained that what a parent does is far more important than what a parent says.

That was the moment Allison acknowledged her true purpose and connected it to her pursuit of health and fitness. During the next 3 months, she became a different person. She never missed another workout. She trained with greater intensity without complaining. She took her daughter for walks in the evening and hikes on the weekends. When asked what it was that helped her connect the dots, Allison said that the conversation we had had finally allowed her to see how her old behaviors and choices were impacting her daughter, who is the most important person in the world to Allison. Allison's number one priority became her health because she saw it as the most powerful way to reach her goals for herself and her child.

Finding and using your purpose as your internal driving force is imperative to changing the metabolic messengers that often trigger your automatic thoughts and behaviors. When you eat or exercise, you secrete a host of metabolic messengers that determine whether you burn fat or store it. Your emotions, beliefs, and thoughts work in a similar fashion to control motivation, energy, drive, and focus.

Having a clearly defined purpose begins the process of change from the inside out and works with food and exercise. Only when the two are in complete alignment have you been successful in mastering the Metabolic Effect.

All metabolic types have difficulty reaching an understanding of their purpose. Muscle burners spend so much time worrying about everything and everyone else that they don't take the time to find out how to take care of themselves. Sugar burners, on the other hand, know what they want, but have trouble figuring out how to achieve it. Mixed burners, as usual, are somewhere in the middle and are often swayed by their immediate circumstances rather than a specific purpose.

Once you know your purpose, write it down. Many of our clients resist writing anything down, but this has the power to make permanent changes in your life. The statement should be in the first person, present tense, and stated as if it is true right now. Perhaps it's something like "I'm lean and fit, and I want to inspire others in my family to see the possibilities that come with body change and optimal health."

This statement may not move you personally, but to the person who wrote it down, it motivates, energizes, and drives him to do whatever it takes. A purpose statement should be so powerful that just the repeating of the phrase elevates the mood and focuses the mind. Once you have your statement, the key is to connect it directly in your head so it aligns with your goals of change.

Now, think back to the Metabolic Spark and Transformation chapters. They helped you understand firsthand how food and exercise choices alter not only metabolic messengers in the body but also the mind. Once you have had this experience, it is easy to see how both the short-term changes and long-term effects of this new lifestyle can impact every area of your life. Once you tie your purpose to this feeling, the force becomes almost unstoppable. We all know that habitual thinking and poor habits often don't disappear overnight. That is where the practice of focus comes in.

Focus

With your purpose and fat-loss goals firmly implanted in your conscious mind, it's time to work on using the metabolic messengers to imprint this same belief into the unconscious mind. This is done through focusing your imagination on exactly what you want. To do so you will use two powerful imagination tools. One is called purpose visualization and the other is called preemptive visualization. Just like the basketball players imagining shooting baskets in their head, you will use these tools both to solidify your purpose and practice your new lifestyle. These are simple techniques and are best done last thing at night and then again first thing in the morning. Together they will begin to wire your conscious and subconscious beliefs together in a way that creates lasting change. Every single time you engage in these practices you will be setting into motion a unique mix of molecular signals that are literally able to imprint this new reality into your brain as if it were really happening. The more you do it, the more effective you become and the more you can create your new reality. We realize this may seem hard to believe, but these practices have been used by athletes and top performers for centuries. You can use these same performance-enhancing techniques to improve your own performance in everyday life.

VISUALIZING YOUR PURPOSE

Remember that the unconscious and conscious minds are different. The conscious mind is very linear, logical, and reasoning. The unconscious mind thinks more in the abstract, and pictures and uses the senses. The more real you can paint the picture in your mind's eye, the better. You want to imagine all possible aspects of something—the way it feels and looks, the color and the texture, the smell and the taste, etc. The more information you give the brain and the more vividly you can imagine the scenario, the better.

Purpose visualization involves you imagining yourself doing something closely tied to your purpose. You want to imagine yourself as if you are standing outside your body watching yourself. A good way to think about this is by watching yourself as if you were watching a movie, yet feeling and sensing everything the main character is going through. The setting here is crucial. You want to imagine yourself in a place that is indicative of the realization of your true purpose. Using some of the examples we gave you above to guide you, here is how you might set up this visualization.

If your major purpose is to be a positive role model for your child, then perhaps you imagine yourself at your daughter's college graduation, meeting her outside after she received her diploma. You hear the sounds and clamoring of people, see all the brightly colored gowns, smell the flowers, and feel the warm spring breeze. Most important, you see yourself, fit, lean, smiling, and happy. Your fit and confident daughter is as proud of you as you are of her. You imagine meeting her friends, feeling their firm handshakes, seeing their warm smiles, and hearing from everyone how warm, friendly, and kind your daughter is to all her friends. You hear others talking about the marathon the two of you will run together in a few weeks. You imagine this in all its detail, down to the minutest—smells, colors, shapes, words, voices, and faces. But most of all, you see yourself there. This is the embodiment of the realization of your purpose. You look, feel, and function like you are young, vibrant, and fit, and so does your daughter.

With this powerful visualization you'll be downloading a very specific and concrete set of instructions to your unconscious mind through metabolic messengers induced by your thoughts. The best time to do this is just before bed as you lie down and are dozing off to sleep. This is a perfect time, a time when the unconscious mind is more receptive and the conscious mind is less intrusive. These techniques should be done daily for as little as a few minutes to as long as you like. This imagined reality will take hold of the automatic workings of the body and start to impact the way you move through your days and alter your metabolic function.

PREEMPTIVE VISUALIZATION

Preemptive visualization is another tool you can use to reprogram your automatic behaviors and beliefs. This technique, directed at the behaviors and scenarios you'll encounter in the day ahead of you, is like the visualization the basketball players used in their mental practice. This works by simply playing the coming day in your head exactly the way you expect it to play out. It is like a mental dress rehearsal and can be extremely powerful in its effects. The technique is simple and takes anywhere from a few seconds to several minutes. We recommend doing this first thing in the morning when you wake up, while you're in the shower, or on your way to work.

Visually walk yourself through the day, starting from where you are at that moment. If you're in the shower, imagine your day from the minute you get out and dry off. See yourself going through all the major events of the day. For example, if you're a stay-at-home mom or dad, perhaps you visualize your day something like this:

"I woke up at six thirty A.M. and worked out before getting the kids up at seven A.M. It's seven fifteen, and I'm eating my first meal of the day—egg whites with Canadian bacon and a piece of fruit. The kids are eating eggs and toast. I make sure the two kids have their schoolwork and lunches packed. I drive them to school at eight and head off with the baby to do errands. At ten A.M. I eat the apple I brought along and a handful of almonds from the stash in my car while the baby has a snack. We head home after visiting my mother. Once the baby eats and goes to sleep, I make myself a salad with sliced chicken, greens, and other veg-etables. I do several loads of laundry and other chores. Before picking up the kids at school, I eat an apple. I drive the kids to their afterschool soccer game. So I'm not tempted by the snacks and sodas for parents and players, I eat a protein bar and drink the water I keep in the car. We go home and I start to prepare dinner while the kids do their homework. I have a large glass of water with fiber so I'm not tempted to nibble. I eat only 10 bites of the mashed potatoes but as much of the roast turkey breast and steamed vegetables as I want. While the older kids clean up, I put the baby in the stroller and my husband and I go for a walk to talk and catch up on the day. If I sit down and watch TV, I will want to eat. When we return, we help the kids with their homework, bathe them, and read bedtime stories together. We turn in by ten thirty."

Or, perhaps you work in an office and you visualize your day something like this: "I wake at six A.M. and drink a cup of black coffee before my workout. I shower, dress, and make a whey protein smoothie with frozen strawberries to drink on the way to work. I restock my briefcase with some protein bars, nuts, and fruit to nibble on around ten thirty, between meetings. At twelve thirty, I go out to lunch with colleagues to a local Mexican place. I drink 2 glasses of water and order a salad right away to avoid the chips. I order chicken fajitas with the grilled vegetables, but tell the waiter no tortillas. I eat 5 bites of the rice and beans. At three thirty I take a break, drink a large cup of green tea, and eat an apple. Since it's raining, I head to the gym after work and walk for 30 minutes on the indoor track and then pedal on the stationary bike for another 30 minutes. Before meeting friends for drinks, I eat a protein bar. We meet and I order sparkling water with lime. At home I make a large salad from vegetables and chicken, already in the fridge, sprinkled with feta cheese and a bit of vinaigrette dressing. I bake a potato in the microwave and eat half, including the skin. I read a book until lights out at ten thirty P.M."

These visualizations are specific, down to the smallest detail. You can make visualizations as general or as simple as you wish. Some clients have successfully used the technique of simply seeing themselves driving to the fitness center after work or packing their gym bag in the morning. They have reported consistently that these imaging techniques improve the likelihood of their actually getting there. One woman found herself pulling into her fitness center only to remember that on that day she had to meet a friend for an early dinner. That is the power of the subconscious mind when you have it working for you.

Sharon: Using Visualizations to Accomplish Fitness Goals

Sixty-two years old and retired, Sharon has always been thin, but once menopause set in she put on a significant amount of fat around her belly. She told us that she's a smoker and suffers from depression, taking four different medications. Sharon's brain chemistry was driving her to want to eat and had sapped her motivation. When she was young, she'd cut back on calories and would lose those few extra pounds that occasionally crept on.

She said she had severe cravings for sweets, coffee, and cigarettes. She had tried Weight Watchers, Jenny Craig, and other weight-loss programs to get rid of that belly fat, but to no avail. Her desire for what she craved only got worse. When we first met with her, Sharon weighed 160 pounds and had 33 percent body fat.

Sharon was a typical muscle burner—thin for most of her life, but with little muscle tone and a less than efficient metabolism.

Sharon began by limiting her bites of starch to 15 at each meal and worked out 3 times a week with an ME outdoor group. Exercising with weights was essential because chemicals from the muscles "spoke" to the rest of her body and helped her brain control her cravings and elevate her mood.

The workout and muscle-burner diet made her feel more balanced, but her cravings remained a challenge. Cups of cocoa and smoothies made with whey protein powder supplied amino acids to build muscle and provide precursors to brain metabolic messengers like serotonin, dopamine, and others for mood changes.

Since she was retired and no longer had a set schedule, we worked out meal and exercise programs for the same times every day. On the days when she wasn't meeting with her ME group, she walked instead. Visualizations became an important part of her new routine as well. Before getting out of bed in the morning, Sharon would visualize the coming day and think about her healthy meals, her workout, and her new lifestyle. In the evenings she would visualize the day in reverse, imagining any areas where she was less than perfect as if she had done it perfectly. She said these visualizations helped her feel less stressed and depressed and more in control and balanced.

During the next 9 months Sharon lost 30 pounds—especially around that troublesome middle area—and 10 percent body fat. Her doctors took her off all of her antidepressant medications except one. She walks daily, attends yoga classes once or twice each week, and does the ME workout twice a week. She has maintained her weight loss for more than 2 years now and describes herself as a different person. She is still working on quitting smoking, but is now in control of her sweet cravings and coffee habit. She credits her success to the combination of a program that used diet, exercise, and behavior modification with an emphasis on visualization as key to her success.

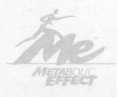

Choice

Once you align your purpose and begin to focus, your metabolic messengers will support your fat-loss goals and influence the choices you make. The nutrition and exercise tools you've been using through the Metabolic Spark and Transformation Stages have already begun this process. And as we've discussed, they also impact your choices directly by altering the neurohormones that make up the molecules of emotion as well as the more direct hormonal influences over fat burning.

Despite the obvious benefit of their influence, you have to continue to make those choices day in and day out to develop the rituals and habits that solidify that metabolic effect. If you don't have a plan, these choices can become overwhelming and can often end with you making no choice at all, which can be just as detrimental as making the wrong choice. If you planned to eat well, but didn't prepare a healthy lunch and find yourself at a fast-food restaurant, what are you going to do? Sure, you can choose not to eat at all, but does this serve your fat-loss goals? That is a strategy in the world of weight loss, but in the world of fat loss you know choosing to skip a meal at lunch will likely send your physiology into a ravenous search for fats and sugar later that night. To avoid this, choose instead to stick to the rules of your metabolic type. Choose the leanest source of meat, perhaps a grilled chicken sandwich without mayo, but with extra lettuce and tomato. Choose to remove the fat-storing bun, using the extra lettuce to make a wrap. Once you learn, practice, and master the techniques of a fat-burning lifestyle, they will become second nature to you. You will be able to control your choices, not the other way around.

Many people resist any attempts at planning and scheduling, but doing so is essential to making the effects of the Metabolic Effect permanent. There are several keys to planning and scheduling that need to be understood. Research shows that as much as we may think we humans are good at multitasking, we're not. We perform much better when we have a defined schedule. Being successful at fat loss means more than making the right choice in the moment; it means setting yourself up to make the right choice ahead of time by using the following steps:

1. Define your purpose.

2. Use purpose visualizations and preemptive visualizations to plant the unconscious seeds of success and belief. Set aside 1 to 10 minutes every day—first thing in the morning when you wake up, while taking a shower, on your way to work or school, or before drifting off to sleep.

3. Plan out everything—meals, your workouts, your shopping lists, and any areas of your life that will present challenges.

4. Take action.

TRACK YOUR PROGRESS

Many of our clients get confused when we tell them to continue to track their progress even after they see dramatic changes in their physiques. Why? Because sometimes we don't realize until it is too late that we've begun to slip back into old self-defeating habits. You need reminders and feedback mechanisms to keep you on the Metabolic Effect path. We have found that the best way to track your progress is by using a body-composition scale, discussed on page 108. But now you'll use it in a different way. Just like an oven timer or seat belt warning in a car, you need a reminder to refocus your attention on what is important. Once you have made your transformation, we suggest you set a trigger body-fat percent. For example, if you have transformed your body and your body fat is now 18 percent, you may want to set your trigger body fat at 20 percent. Once a week at the same time, perhaps Sunday morning before you eat anything, you'll use your body fat-scale to check your percentage. This will reinforce you in maintaining your 18 percent level. If one morning, however, you step on the scale and it shows that your body fat is at 21 percent, that's an all-out warning sign that it's time to refocus your purpose and get back to the basics that keep you in fat-burning mode. Are you eating more than your allotted bites of starches? Are you giving in to those food cravings? Not sleeping enough? Skipping workouts? You have the knowledge and the tools to refocus your goals and reassess how to achieve them.

This body-fat trigger should be a number close to where you are now. You don't want to wait until you have gained 10 percent body fat to take action. We suggest this number be no more than 2 to 3 percent from the lowest body composition you achieved. Once you hit this number it should be like an alarm going off in your head that your body is moving out of the Metabolic Effect and you should immediately be asking why. Have you stopped doing your workouts? Are you walking less? Have you been drinking too much alcohol? This strategy is employed by all of our clients who have been able to attain and maintain optimal body change over the long run.

Once you've established your trigger body-fat percentage, you should construct a plan to get you moving back in the right direction. We call this the emergency-aid kit and it's used to give the metabolism an extra boost to get it back to where it needs to be. The first thing you need to do before enacting a plan is to have a good understanding of what has gone wrong. Answering these five questions will help you pinpoint where the issues are coming from and what to focus on to get back on track.

1. Do I have a schedule and stick to it?

2. Have I been sleeping at least 7 to 9 hours a night?

3. Have I been managing my stress appropriately?

4. Have I been without hunger, low energy, or excessive cravings?

5. Am I minimizing my intake of alcohol, caffeine, and stimulants?

If you answer no to any of these questions, then you have a clear idea about what you need to do to get back on track. Humans thrive on regimented schedules and always function better when they have a plan to follow. When thrown off schedule, pick up where you left off or create a new schedule that reflects your new circumstances and takes into account your meals, exercise, relaxation time, sleep, etc.

Remember, sleep is your hormonal reset button. Without sleep you'll wake with higher cortisol levels and therefore crave more sweets and fatty foods as well as seek out caffeine and other stimulants. Both too much sleep and too little sleep can get you in trouble as far as your hormonal fat burning is concerned. A good schedule starts with good sleep. If you are unable to sleep, you need to work hard to figure out what is causing it. Above all else, work to put yourself back to sleep. Alcohol, caffeine, stress, illness, and lifestyle changes like having a new baby in the house or losing a job can all impact sleep. Eating a balanced metabolic diet and exercising are two of the most powerful sleep aids you have. If you've tried everything else and still can't sleep, stay awake the entire night and next day, setting your bedtime at the time you would like to sleep. This technique can often restore a healthy sleep pattern. Remember—don't consume caffeine, sugar, or other stimulants to make it through the day. Instead use food and exercise to manage your energy levels.

If you're under a great amount of stress, both your sleep schedule and daily routine are likely to be affected. Again, this is the time when your nutritional and exercise habits should be more, not less, regimented. Focusing on what you can control rather than on what you can't control will help you regain your metabolic balance more quickly.

Use both your purpose visualization and your preemptive visualization to counteract stress and refocus.

If you notice that your energy, hunger, or cravings are getting the best of you, then your issues likely have to do with metabolic imbalances caused by shifts in diet or exercise habits. This often occurs after a long vacation or celebration where you indulged just a little too much. You would be surprised by what just one weekend of overeating and overdrinking can do. We often see people return from a honeymoon, high school reunion, or friend's wedding and just can't seem to get back on track. This is a time to refocus. Immediately start eating according to your metabolic type to get those fat-burning hormones activated. Return to weight training and walking as soon as possible. Practice your visualizations and revisit your purpose statement as frequently as necessary to get you refocused.

It's easy to fall back into old habits. At first, one or two nights out for cocktails or a few cups of coffee may not affect your metabolism, but stay on that path and the fatigue, lack of motivation, and depression or anxiety will return. Look at what you've been doing for the last few weeks. Drinking a glass of wine with dinner? Eating more than those allotted bites of certain foods? Enjoying those Reward Meals 3 times a week instead of 1? Remember that food and beverages are information for the body and that every single time you eat or drink you are sending metabolic signals that either serve or hinder your goals. Once you recognize the problem, make the changes that worked for you in the past.

Here's a quick guide for restarting your metabolic engine and getting you back on track as quickly as possible. Begin on a day—usually the weekend—when you have some free time.

1. Walk for 1 hour. During this walk mentally formulate an action plan for refocusing your efforts.

2. Clean your house of all the foods that are not serving your goals and make sure your surroundings are neat and organized. This immediately makes you feel in control.

3. Make a shopping list and go shopping (make sure you go on a full stomach).

4. Prepare all your food for the coming week anticipating exactly what your days will be like, what you will need for meals and snacks, and what you will carry them in. Prep, cook, and store food in plastic containers so they're ready for the week.

5. Schedule your workouts for the week. Write down the days and times on your calendar.

6. Get everything organized for the next day. Pack your gym bag and have your food ready to go.

7. Eat an early dinner and relax by reading, taking a hot bath, or chatting with a friend.

8. Review your purpose statement.

9. Do your purpose visualization just before going to bed.

10. On waking in the morning do your preemptive visualization by thinking about the coming day in all its detail and seeing all the important events unfold in a way that serves you and your goals.

As you progress, you'll see that the ME Diet is more than just an exercise and nutrition program, but also a wonderful way of life. To benefit from the ME Diet, you have to implement and practice all that you've learned in these pages. It will take time and effort to master the Metabolic Effect, but once you do, you'll wonder how you ever lived any other way.

ACKNOWLEDGMENTS

We would like to thank the people without whom this book wouldn't exist.

To Dr. Joseph Teta, grandfather and doctor, for steering us toward such a fulfilling profession. Thank you for your guidance.

To our parents, Jim and Joyce Teta, thank you for believing in us from day one and for your unconditional love and unwavering support.

To our older brother Kimo, who we always look up to and who pushed us to be great. Thank you for taking care of us.

To our sister Jodi, who has consistently supported us, believed in us, and taught us what it means to sacrifice for others.

To John Stevens, our adopted brother, closest family friend, and the genius behind the Metabolic Effect brand. Everyone should be so lucky to have a friend and business partner with your genius, passion, and generosity.

To our amazing wives, Jill Coleman and Jillian Sarno, who are brilliant health-care providers, personal trainers, and people. You are both so beautiful and we love you so much. Your feedback and counsel on this book have been immeasurable.

To Ronnie Baldwin and Gary Leake, our best friends and training partners for years, who have taught us so much about fitness and keep us laughing. Thank you for your support, expertise, and willingness to help no matter what. You are amazing friends and have always been our role models for living the fat-loss lifestyle.

To our nieces and nephews, Alisa, Quentin, Lili, Soul, and Zen, for reminding us to stay in the moment and love each other.

To Linda Pallazotto, Jay Sloatman, Julie Sutton, Inci Brown, Claudia Peterson, Hisham Barakat, Claudine Legault, and Ginny Weiler, for generosity beyond our imaginations. Your love and support have made a real difference in our lives.

To Gaby Scaritt, for working with us on this book from the very beginning and helping us get it off the ground.

To J. J. Virgin, Mark Smith, and Linda Lizotte, for believing in our work from the beginning.

To Frank Devin, for recognizing the potential in our work and teaching us about business.

To Jaclyn Chasse, our favorite New Hampshire naturopathic physician, thank you for seeing the value in our work.

To Chris Clodfelter, MMA fighter and personal trainer, for your excitement and passion for the Metabolic Effect system from day one. We value your friendship.

To Esther Blum, for believing in this project and guiding us to make it happen. You have been an angel and we are so grateful for your showing up in our lives.

To our agent, Celeste Fine, beautiful and brilliant beyond belief. We feel so lucky to have you in our corner.

To Harriet Bell, our amazing writer, who took our words and ideas and made us sound so smart. Thank you for your guidance on all aspects of this project.

Thank you to our amazing photographer Lisa Brewer and top-notch fitness models Obi Obadike, Jill Coleman, Jillian Sarno, Gary Leake, and Rebecca Schwartz.

To Loren Cordain, Alwyn Cosgrove, Christian Finn, Charles Staley, Barry Sears, Joe Pizzorno, T. S. Wiley, Jeffrey Bland, Bill Philips, Joseph Mercola, Robert Crayhon, Mark Houston, and Bruce Lipton. While we don't know all of you personally, we would like to acknowledge your contributions to our field and your influence on our work.

To Jack LaLanne and Albert Beckles, for helping us realize the secret to the fountain of youth.

To the Winston-Salem, North Carolina, family of Metabolic Effect participants and the YWCA and YMCAs that run our programs. Thank you for all your support and enthusiasm.

To the field of medically trained naturopathic physicians, the two hundred Metabolic Effect certified trainers who run our workouts at gyms and in parks all over the country, and to the thousands of people who participate in Metabolic Effect workouts. Thank you for helping create sustainable health and fitness in yourself, your clients, and your patients.

Finally, to all our teachers, coaches, mentors, and counselors through the years, thank you for helping us find our calling and life's work.

RESOURCES
FOODS, SUPPLEMENTS, AND EQUIPMENT

PROTEIN BARS

Not all protein bars are equal. Many of them have too many carbs. Here are the ones we suggest and that are available online or at supermarkets and health food stores.

Glucobalance bars (www.metaboliceffect.com)
Sugar burners: Diabetone bar
Mixed burners: Glucobalance peanut butter chocolate bars or
    Diabetone bars
Muscle burners: UltraLean Crispy Rice and UltraLean Spice bars
CocoChia bars (www.livingfuel.com/CocoChia-Snack-Fuel-Bars.
    aspx)
thinkThin (www.thinkproducts.com/thin-bars.php)
Zone bars and Balance bars (www.balance.com)
Atkins bars (www.atkins.com)

PROTEIN POWDERS

ME The Meal (www.metaboliceffect.com)
ME The Meal DF/dairy free/vegetarian (www.metaboliceffect.com)

Jay Robb, available at Whole Foods and Vitamin Shoppe
Muscle Milk Naturals, available at GNC and Vitamin Shoppe

FIBER

ME Fiber Complex (www.metaboliceffect.com)
Apple pectin, available at most health food stores
Guar gum, available at most health food stores

VEGGIE/FRUIT COMPLEXES

ME Recovery Reds and ME Recovery Greens
(www.metaboliceffect.com)

COCOA POWDERS

Equal Exchange organic baking cocoa (http://www.equalexchange.
    coop/cocoa)
Rapunzel organic cocoa (www.rapunzel.com)
Raw Choice organic cocoa (www.therawchoice.com)

ALTERNATIVE SWEETENERS

Erythritol: ZSweet (www.zsweet.com)
Sweet Simplicity (www.sweetsimplictysweetener.com)
Xylitol: Polysweet (www.xylitolnow.com)
XyloSweet (www.xlear.com)
Truvia and Purevia, available in markets and health food stores

SUPPLEMENTS

For enhanced fat loss from www.metaboliceffect.com:
ME Metabolic Complex: metabolically formulated multivitamin
ME Fat Burner Complex: nonstimulating fat-loss aid

ME High-Potency Omega-3: concentrated omega-3 blend
ME Recovery C: high-potency vitamin C for workout recovery

EQUIPMENT

For weights and benches, we use and recommend the PowerBlock dumbbell system. It's a unique adjustable dumbbell that can take the place of a whole weight room of dumbbells yet takes up the floor space of only one pair (www.metaboliceffect.com).

Tanita body-fat scales that measure muscle mass, fat percentage, water percentage, and weight among others (www.metaboliceffect.com).

Vita-Mix blenders are the most powerful blenders available. Ideal for protein shakes, healthy fruit smoothies, quick soups, and vegetable juices (www.vitamix.com).

Xiser is a portable ergonomically correct sprint trainer. This unit can be kept at home or at the office for quick-burst workouts that effectively mimic sprint training. It is a great adjunct to a fat-loss lifestyle (www.metaboliceffect.com).

Polar heart-rate monitors are for those who want to incorporate heart-rate monitoring into their workouts (www.polarusa.com).

Magic Bullet is a great portable mixer for home, office, and traveling. Recommended for those on the go who want a small but powerful mixer for protein shakes and smoothies (www.buythebullet.com).

SELECTED BIBLIOGRAPHY

Bell, G. J., Syrotuik, D., et al. "Effect of Concurrent Strength and Endurance Training on Skeletal Muscle Properties and Hormone Concentrations in Humans." *European Journal of Applied Physiology* 81, no. 5 (2000): 418–427.

Djurhuus, C. B., Gravholt, C. H., et al. "Additive Effects of Cortisol and Growth Hormone on Regional and Systemic Lipolysis in Humans." *American Journal of Physiology* 286 (2004): E488–E494.

Gladden, L. B. "Lactate Metabolism: A New Paradigm for the Third Millennium." *Journal of Physiology* 558, no. 1 (2004): 5–30.

Jacks, D. E., Sowash, J., et al. "Effect of Exercise at Three Exercise Intensities on Salivary Cortisol." *Journal of Strength and Conditioning Research* 16, no. 2 (2002): 286–289.

Lin, H., Wang, S. W., et al. "Stimulatory Effect of Lactate on Testosterone Production by Rat Leydig Cells." *Journal of Cellular Biochemistry* 83, no. 1 (2001): 147–154.

Lindeberg, S., Jönsson, T., et al. "A Paleolithic Diet Improves Glucose Tolerance More Than a Mediterranean Diet in Individuals with Ischaemic Heart Disease." *Diabetologia* 50, no. 9 (2007): 1795–1807.

McMurray, R. G., and A. C. Hackney. "Interactions of Metabolic Hormones, Adipose Tissue and Exercise." *Sports Medicine* 35, no. 5 (2005): 393–412.

Melanson, E. L., P. S. MacLean, and J. O. Hill. "Exercise Improves Fat Metabolism in Muscle but Does Not Increase 24-H Fat Oxidation." *Exercise and Sport Sciences Reviews* 37, no. 2 (2009): 93–101.

Osterberg, K. L., and C. L. Melby. "Effect of Acute Resistance Exercise on Postexercise Oxygen Consumption and Resting Metabolic Rate in Young Women." *International Journal of Sport Nutrition and Exercise Metabolism* 10, no. 1 (2000): 71–81.

Ottosson, M., Lönnroth, P., et al. "Effect of Cortisol and Growth Hormone on Lipolysis in Human Adipose Tissue." *Journal of Clinical Endocrinology and Metabolism* 85, no. 2 (2000): 799–803.

Pedersen, B. K., Åkerström, T. C. A., et al. "Role of Myokines in Exercise and Metabolism." *Journal of Applied Physiology* 103, no. 3 (2007): 1093–1098.

Pedersen, B. K., Steensberg, A., et al. "Searching for the Exercise Factor: Is Il-6 a Candidate?" *Journal of Muscle Research and Cell Motility* 24, nos. 2–3 (2003): 113–119.

Schuenke, M. D., R. P. Mikat, and J. M. McBride. "Effect of an Acute Period of Resistance Exercise on Excess Post-Exercise Oxygen Consumption: Implications for Body Mass Management." *European Journal of Applied Physiology* 86, no. 5 (2002): 411–417.

Scott, C. "Misconceptions About Aerobic and Anaerobic Energy Expenditure." *Journal of the International Society of Sports Nutrition* 2, no. 2 (2005): 32–37.

Stewart, A. D., and W. J. Hannan. "Prediction of Fat and Fat-Free Mass in Male Athletes Using Dual X-Ray Absorptiometry As the Reference Method." *Journal of Sports Sciences* 18, no. 4 (2000): 263–274.

Teta, J. "Exercise Is Medicine: The Anti-Inflammatory Effects of High

Intensity Exercise," *Townsend Letter for Doctors and Patients,* November 2006.

Teta, J., and K. Teta. "Hormonal Weight Loss: Is There Such a Thing As the 'Metabolic Effect?'" *Townsend Letter for Doctors and Patients,* February/March 2007.

Teta J., and K. Teta. "New Perspectives on Insulin: Contributing Influences on Body Fat and Insulin Resistance." *Townsend Letter for Doctors and Patients,* December 2008.

Tomas, E., Kelly, M., et al. "Metabolic and Hormonal Interactions between Muscle and Adipose Tissue." *Proceedings of the Nutrition Society* 63 (2004): 381–385.

Trapp, E. G., Chisholm, D. J., et al. "The Effects of High-Intensity Intermittent Exercise Training on Fat Loss and Fasting Insulin Levels of Young Women." *International Journal of Obesity* 32 (2008): 684–691.

THE METABOLIC EFFECT

If you'd like to learn more about *The New ME Diet* and the Metabolic Effect, here are some additional resources:

www.metaboliceffect.com
www.metaboliceffect.wordpress.com (blog)
www.facebook.com/pages/Winston-Salem-NC/Metabolic-
   Effect/79608796892
http://twitter.com/metaboliceffect
www.naturopathichealthclinic.com
http://www.youtube.com/user/metaboliceffect (see how exercises
   are done)

For information on where to find gyms, trainers, or group exercise instructors that offer the ME program, visit our Web site.

If you own a gym or are a trainer who would like to add our program to your center, please contact us at:

Metabolic Effect Inc.
2522 Reynolda Road
Winston-Salem, NC 27106
contactme@metaboliceffect.com
1 (877) 88-ME FIT, Ext. 81

INDEX

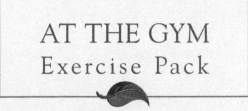

AT THE GYM
Exercise Pack

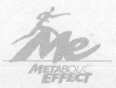

BACK HYBRIDS

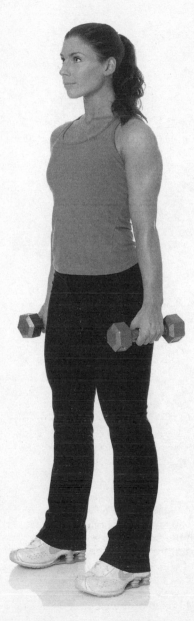

1. Squat/Row: With weights by your sides, sit backward as you lower your body into a squat. Then, pause at the bottom while pulling the weights up to the side of your waist. Lower the weights and return to standing. Repeat 12 times.

1

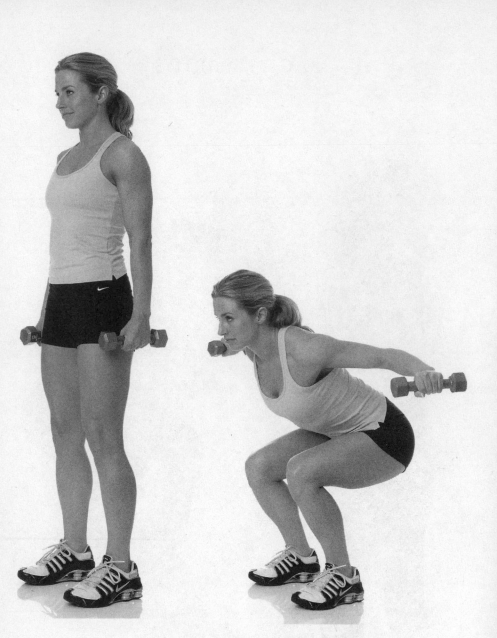

2. Squat/Bent-over Fly: With weights by your sides, sit backward as you lower your body into a squat. Then, pause at the bottom while lifting the weights to the sides of the body, keeping your elbows slightly bent and squeezing your shoulder blades together. Return to standing and repeat 12 times. Arms should be perpendicular to your torso with a slight bend at the elbow.

3. Static Squat/Row/Fly:
With weights by your sides, hold yourself in a squatting position with your weights hanging just in front of your knees. Then pull the weights straight up and even with your waist. Lower them and bring them out to the sides with your arms perpendicular to your torso, keeping your elbows slightly bent. Repeat these two movements in a continuous motion 12 times.

4. In Place Lunge/Row: Standing with your feet together and holding dumbbells by your sides, take a big step forward with your right leg and drop your back knee straight down toward the ground. Your front knee should fall in line with your front ankle, creating a 90-degree angle between your upper and lower leg. Lean forward at the waist and pull the weights up by squeezing your shoulder blades together and bending your arms. The weights should be even with your belly button. Relax the arms and then push back forcefully on the front heel to return to a standing position before repeating the movement on the other side. Do 6 repetitions on each leg for 12 rows total.

CHEST HYBRIDS

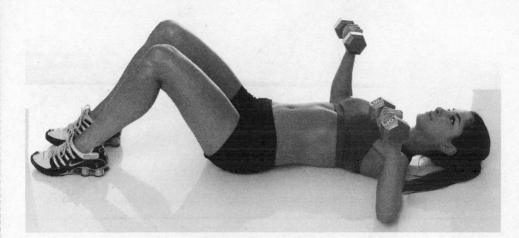

1. Chest Press/Crunch: Lying on your back, press the weights up toward the ceiling while lifting your shoulder blades off the floor and contracting your abs. Hold this position for a count of 2, release, and repeat 12 times.

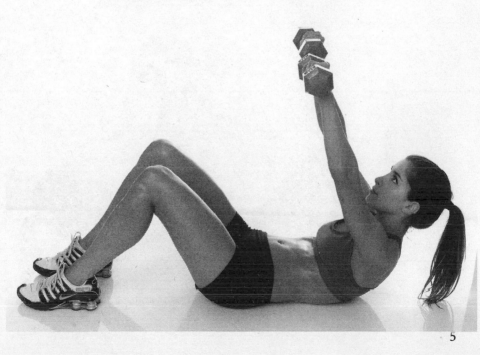

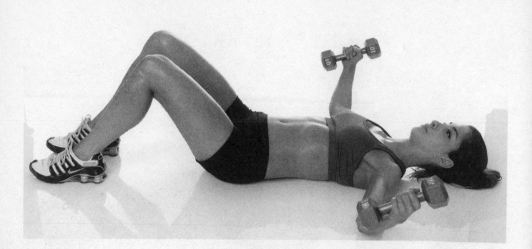

2. Chest Fly/Crunch: Lying on your back, bring the weights out toward the sides of the body in an arcing motion until they meet in front of you with arms slightly bent and dumbbells touching. Squeeze the weights together, as if you are giving someone a hug, and lift your shoulder blades off the floor at the same time and contract your abs. Hold this position for a count of 2, release, and repeat 12 times.

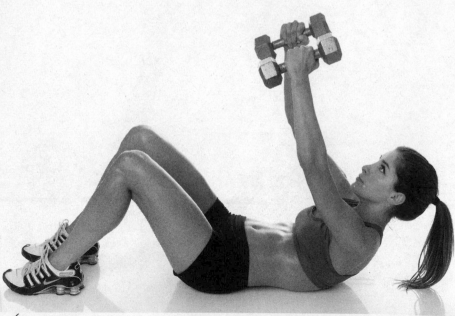

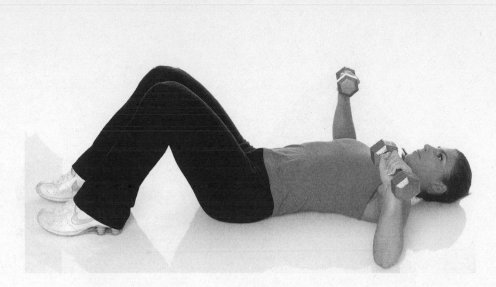

3. Chest Press/Chest Fly: Lying on your back, press the weights straight up toward the ceiling, then slowly lower the weights by bending the elbows slightly and, in a wide arcing pattern, let the arms move out to the sides of the body. Bring the weights back up in the same arcing pattern (fly). When the weights are at the top, lower them straight down. Repeat the entire movement 12 times.

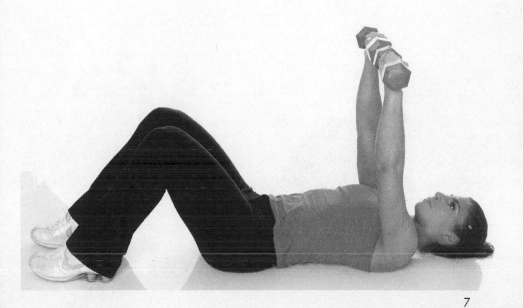

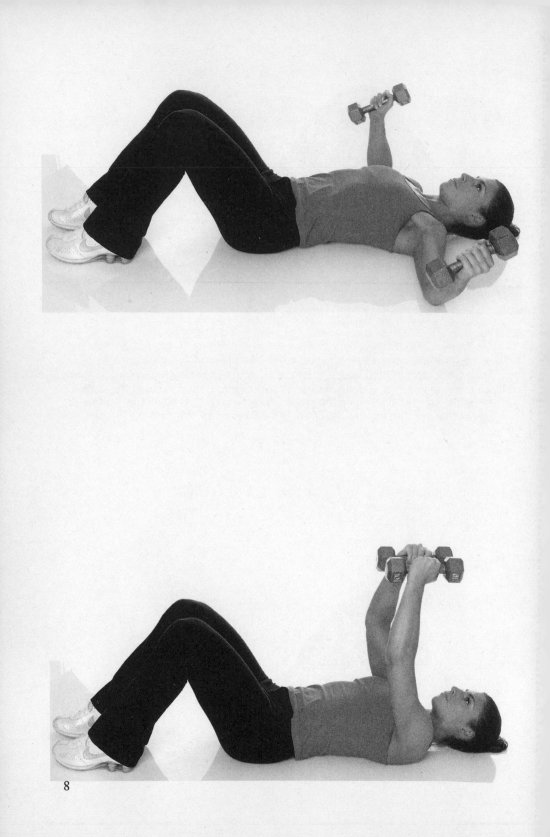

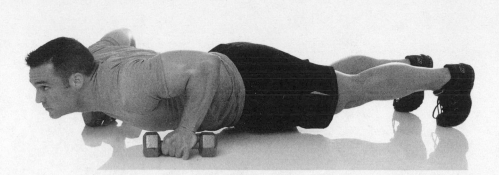

4. Push-up/Row: In a push-up position (on the knees or the toes) with the dumbbells in your hands, do a push-up by lowering your chest toward the floor. As you push back up, row one weight to the side of the body. Lower that weight and repeat the push-up, then row the other weight. Continue alternating, doing a push-up and a row on one side followed by a push-up and then a row on the other side for a total of 12 repetitions.

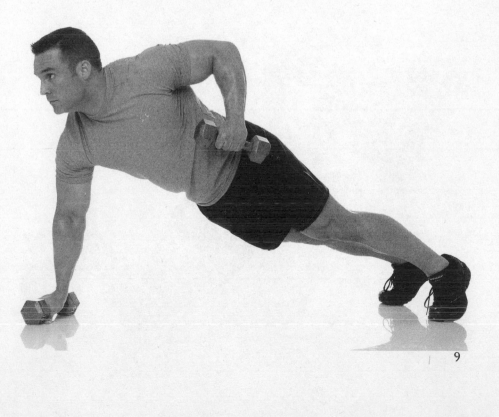

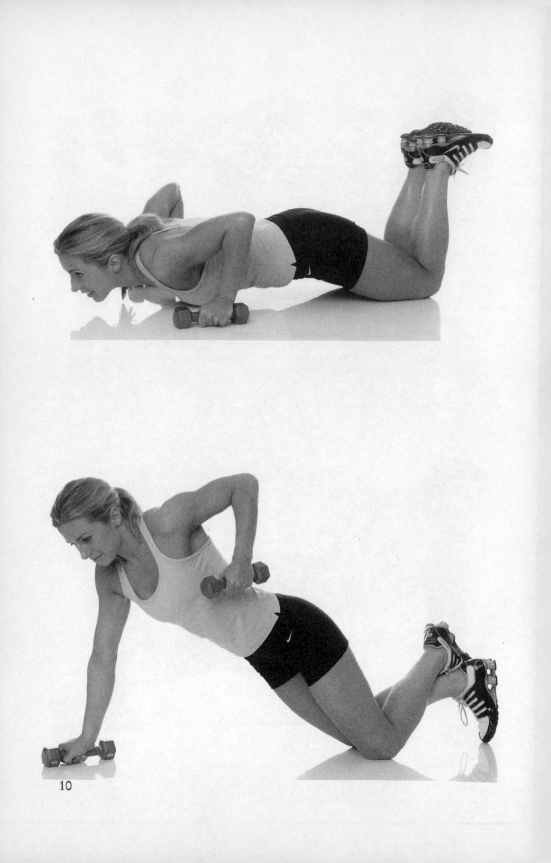

ARM HYBRIDS

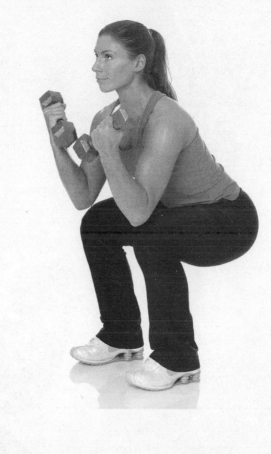

1. Squat/Curl: With the weights by your sides, sit down in a squat position. Hold the position and curl the weights up to your shoulders at the same time. Return the arms to the side and stand back up. Repeat 12 times.

2. Curl/Extension: Holding yourself in a squat position with the weights by your sides, curl the weights to the front of the body, and then in a controlled motion bring the elbows close to the sides of the body while keeping the arms bent. Extend the arms up and back into a tricep extension. Repeat the movement by alternating between the curl and extension 12 times, staying in a squat position throughout.

3. Row/Extension: In a squat position, let the weights hang straight down. Pull the weights up to the waist while squeezing the shoulder blades. Without taking tension off the shoulder blades, straighten the elbows so that the weights are behind the body in a tricep extension. Reverse. Repeat the entire movement 12 times.

4. Lunge/Curl/Press: Step into a lunge position and curl the weights from the sides of the body to shoulder level, then press the weights straight overhead. Lower the weights to your sides and push back to a standing position. Lunge on the other side and repeat the entire movement 12 times (6 lunges on each leg and 12 curl/press).

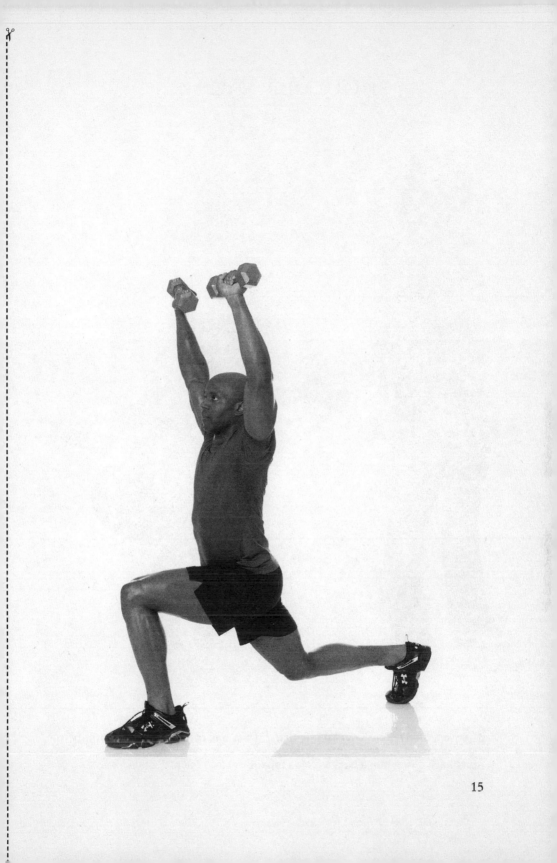

SHOULDER HYBRIDS

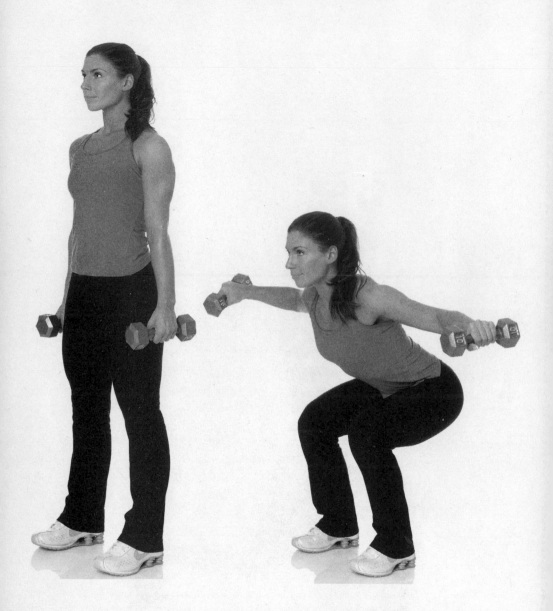

1. Squat/Side Raise: Squat down, then lift the weights out to the sides of the body, keeping the elbows slightly bent. Then bring the arms back down, stand back up, and repeat the movement 12 times.

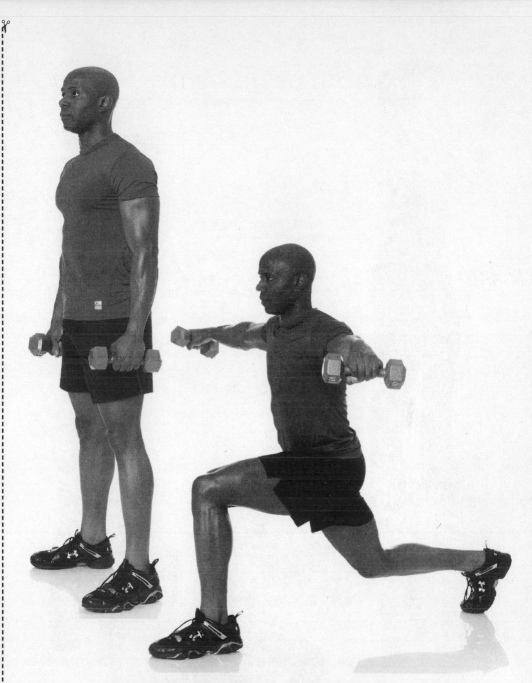

2. Lunge/Side Raise: Step into a lunge position and then lift the weights straight out to the sides of the body, keeping the elbows bent and not lifting past shoulder height. Bring the arms down to the sides of the body. Push back to standing and repeat on the opposite side. Repeat this entire movement 12 times (6 lunges on each leg and 12 side raises).

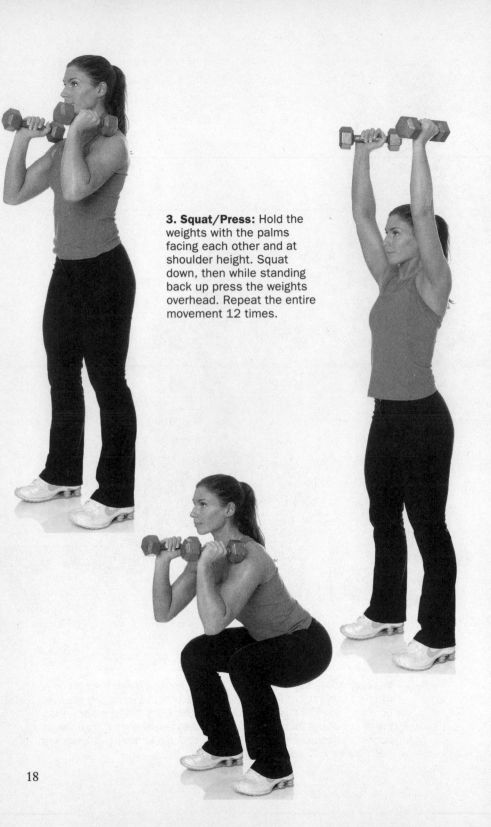

3. Squat/Press: Hold the weights with the palms facing each other and at shoulder height. Squat down, then while standing back up press the weights overhead. Repeat the entire movement 12 times.

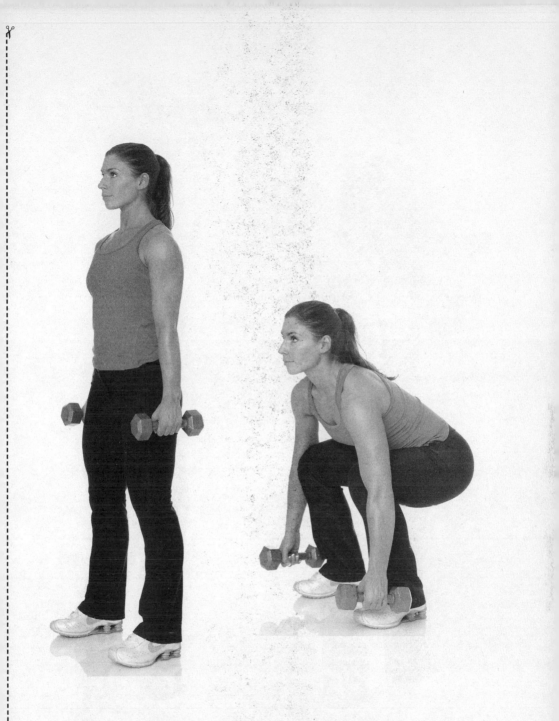

4. Dead Lift/Curl/Press: With the weights by the sides of your body, squat until the weights touch the ground. As you stand up, curl the weights, then press them overhead. Repeat 12 times.

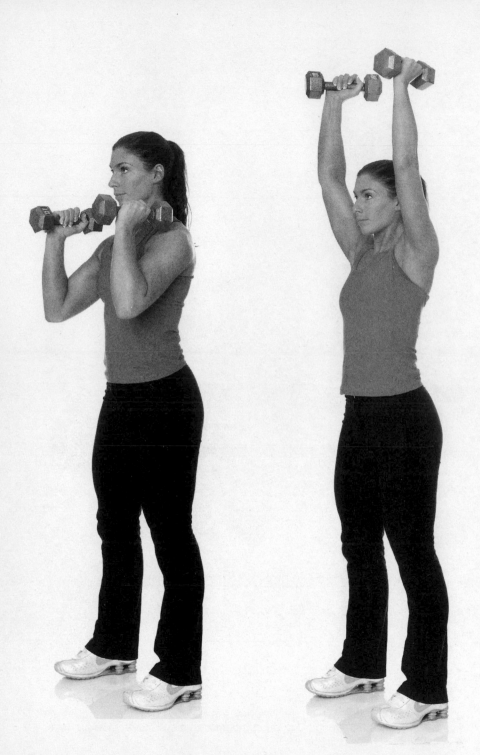

SUPERSETS
Pairing 1: Push-ups and Rows

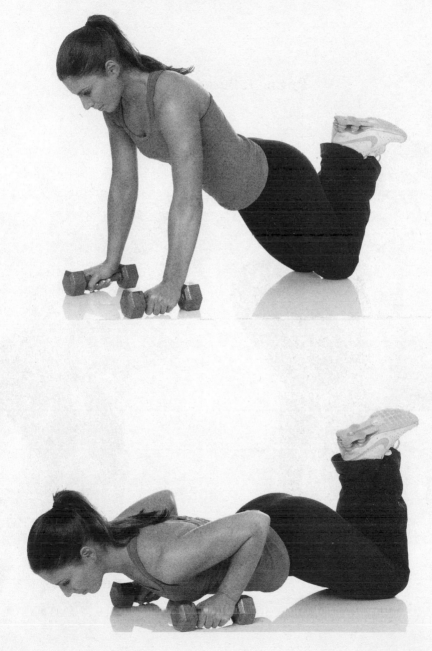

Pairing 1: Push-ups and Rows

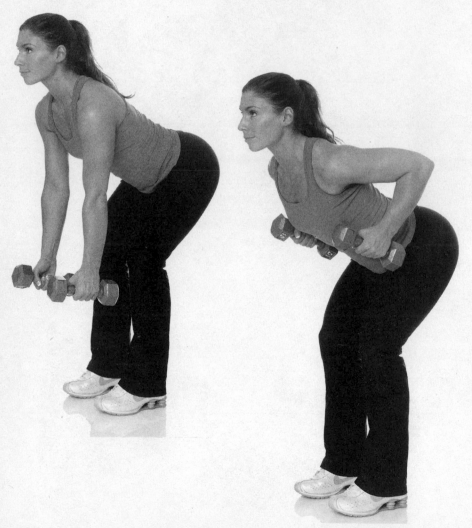

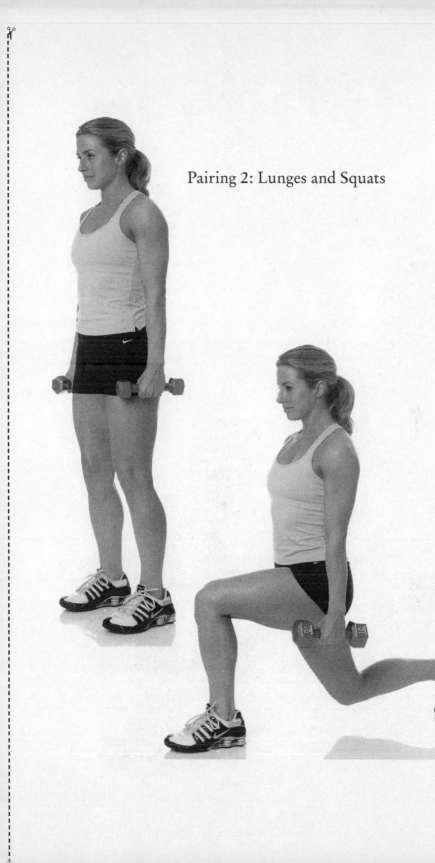

Pairing 2: Lunges and Squats

Pairing 2: Lunges and Squats

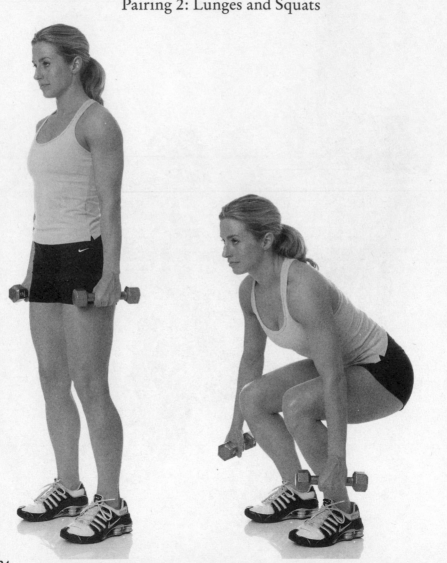

Pairing 3: Biceps Curls and Tricep Dips

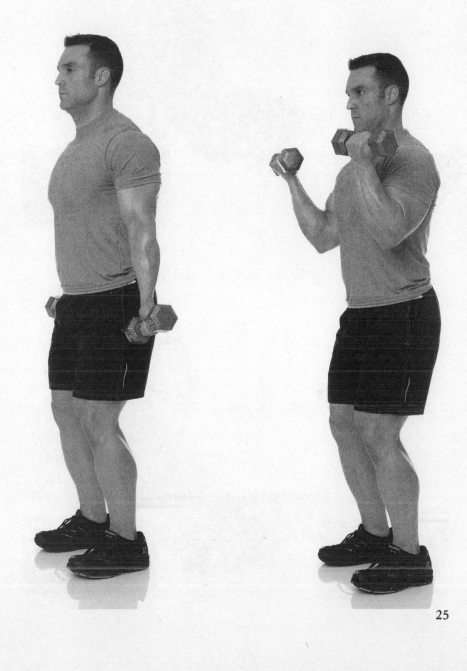

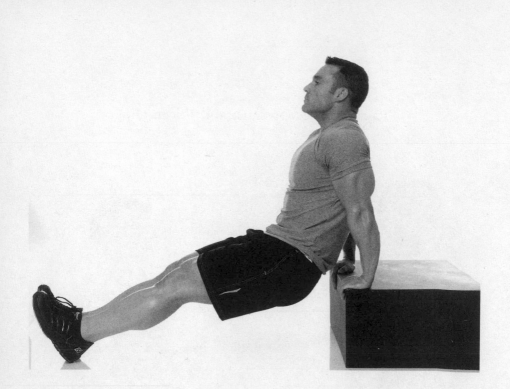

Pairing 3: Biceps Curls and Tricep Dips

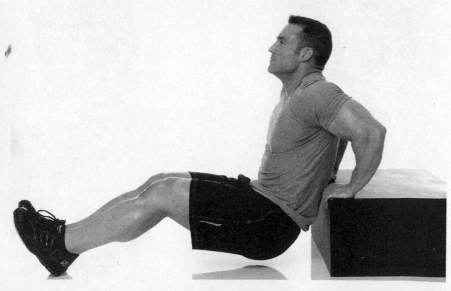

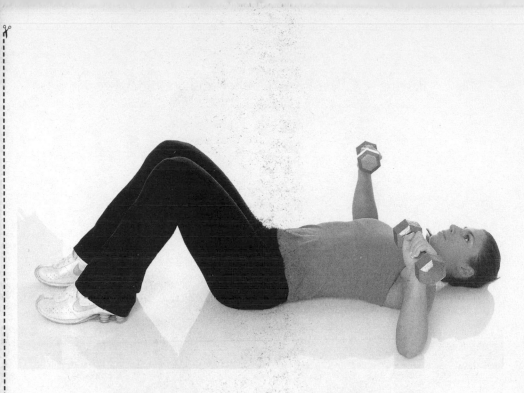

Pairing 4: Chest Press/Crunch and Shoulder Press

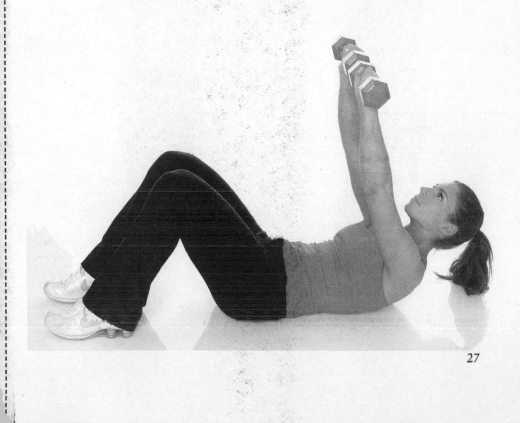

Pairing 4: Chest Press/Crunch and Shoulder Press

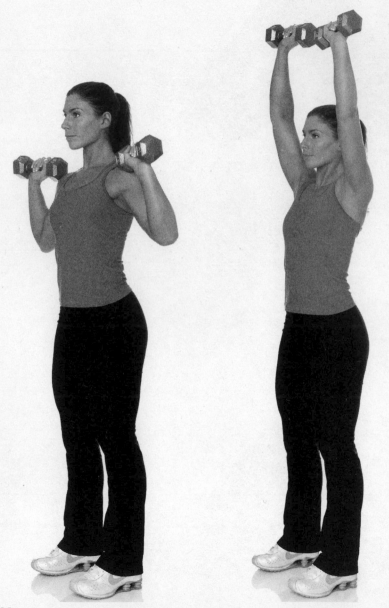